HEALING FROM

UNEXPLAINED SECONDARY INFERTILITY

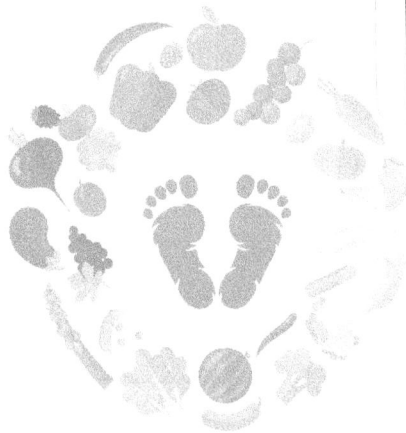

PRACTICAL TIPS FROM A NUTRITIONIST WHO OVERCAME
10 YEARS OF UNEXPLAINED SECONDARY INFERTILITY
TO CONCEIVE NATURALLY AND GIVE BIRTH AT AGE 44

CATHERINE GARNEY

I dedicate this book to my beautiful rainbow child Jenah who inspired this book, and to all rainbow babies and much hoped for babies out there waiting to be born.

Also, to my family for supporting me while I pursued this crazy idea of writing a book.

Contents

Introduction

As I sit here in March of 2021 watching my beautiful miracle daughter play with her toys, I am filled with so much love and gratitude. Three years ago, I never thought I would be here. In fact, during my 10-year journey with secondary infertility, I never imagined that I would be so blessed.

Three years ago, I delivered a workshop in my local town on optimising fertility. As a nutritionist who was also struggling with infertility, I had a great deal of knowledge to share so I felt it would be a good idea to run a workshop. This is because I really wanted to help others by passing on the knowledge I had learned as a practitioner. Although the workshop went well, I felt like an imposter afterwards. I felt I had no right to be running a workshop on optimising fertility when I still hadn't held on to a pregnancy myself. Although I had researched everything I could about fertility from a practitioner's point of view, I still hadn't made it past seven weeks of pregnancy. This was my issue. I didn't have a problem conceiving, even with my advancing age. It was holding on to the pregnancies that were my problem. Over the 10 years I battled with secondary infertility, I suffered multiple miscarriages and chemical pregnancies, which are very early pregnancy losses usually between four and five weeks. I lost count of how many losses I had in the end but would have been over 17.

To find out that I was pregnant naturally at age 43, after 10 years of infertility and recurrent pregnancy loss, was truly a miracle to me. This was because by this point, I accepted that it was unlikely to happen.

At age 40, we had our only round of in vitro fertilisation (IVF) as we only qualified for one round because of my age, and we couldn't afford to fund it ourselves. Despite the procedure being successful, it sadly ended in a miscarriage at six weeks. At my post-IVF review meeting with my fertility doctor, I was told that my eggs were too old and that my only option was to go down the donor route.

I didn't want to do this, so at age 41 I let go of my dreams, well not totally because anyone who has experienced infertility knows that letting go is hard to do. There is always a "what if?". It is never truly over until it becomes physically impossible to get pregnant, like reaching menopause, which might not have been that far away for me. I left it up to the universe to decide if I was ever going to have a baby. I couldn't completely let go though, so at the beginning of each week I wrote in my weekly goals journal:

"I would love to get pregnant if it was safe and possible for me to do so."

At age 43 and after two years of regularly writing this as a goal in my journal, I finally became pregnant and carried my daughter to term with no major issues. Maybe my baby was waiting for the right time, the right moment, to enter our lives. She only showed up when everything in my life was aligned. I truly believe this.

What is infertility?

Infertility is when you have been trying unsuccessfully to get pregnant for 12 months or more, or six months or more if you are over the age of 35. If you are lucky, testing will identify a reason. However, many couples unfortunately don't find out a reason, and they receive the diagnosis of unexplained infertility. When you receive the label of infertility, especially unexplained, it is difficult not to blame yourself and think that there is something wrong with you. Many times, infertility is really just an imbalance, not a disease. It is a sign that something is slightly off, and not in a healthy balance, which is creating an internal environment that is not optimal for conceiving and carrying a baby to term. It is a sign you are not quite ready to have a baby. You may feel in your heart and mind that you are ready, but physically, you are not ready.

Hormone imbalances can contribute to many cases of unexplained infertility. The most common are low progesterone, estrogen dominance, low testosterone and adrenal or thyroid dysfunction. Additional factors may be issues with methylation and folate metabolism, autoimmune conditions driven by poor gut health, and nutritional deficiencies. These causes can be remedied in time for many individuals.

Many couples do not have the chance to investigate these options, as they are told that IVF is their only option. However, this is not always the case. I recommend that every couple that is considering IVF takes four months off trying to conceive to optimise their fertility prior to the procedure. It is also worth getting further testing done with a fertility practitioner, see what comes up and work to address any imbalances as much as possible before going down the IVF route. This could significantly increase your chances of success.

Four months preconception plan

Four months before you start trying to conceive is when you and your husband or partner's health should be at its most optimal. This will increase your chances of conceiving and giving birth to a healthy baby. This is because it takes approximately 100 days for an egg follicle to mature and around 116 days for sperm to be produced. This is a crucial window of opportunity and if your health is not optimal during this time, then it will affect the health of the sperm and egg, which will make it more challenging to conceive.

The four-month preconception period is an opportunity to address any chronic health issues in both of you that could be affecting your pregnancy success. This could include:

- Improving diet

- Addressing nutritional deficiencies (especially if you have recently stopped taking the oral contraceptive pill)

- Managing stress

- Checking hormone levels and addressing hormone imbalances

- Optimising gut health and rebuilding the gut microbiome

- Investigating allergies and food intolerances, which may cause inflammation in the body

- Supporting detoxification

- Addressing any chronic infections.

A four-month break gives you a chance to have a reset and address any issues that may be holding you back. I know this is really hard to do when you are so desperate for a baby and you feel that your time is running out, but believe me, it can be just what you need to make a difference. I did this a few times during my fertility journey and felt so much better for it, both physically and mentally. If you want to see positive changes occur in your life, it is important to do things differently. Change rarely occurs if we continue doing the same thing over and over again.

What many couples don't realise is that there is an entire world of options to try outside the general advice from their GP or fertility specialist. Many feel that IVF and other fertility treatments are their only option and when IVF is unsuccessful, they run out of options and lose hope.

So why did I write this book? To be honest, I kept thinking about writing it, but then I kept talking myself out of it, saying to myself that no one was going to listen to me and who was I anyway. However, the universe kept giving me little nudges and signs that I needed to do this, such as information on book writing courses dropping into my Facebook feed and business audiobooks, literally screaming at me to write this book.

Whenever I tried to talk myself out of writing this book, I kept thinking of the people I want to help:

- The heartbroken couple frantically searching the internet and forums for advice on how to get pregnant or maintain a pregnancy.

- The couple, who have been told that their only option is IVF and are concerned about the potential cost of the procedure.

- The woman who has been told that she has low AMH levels and is upset that her window of fertility is decreasing.

- The woman who has suffered another miscarriage, and no one knows why they keep happening.

- The couple who cannot afford fertility treatment and are searching the internet for a miracle treatment.

- The woman who feels out of balance but doesn't know what to do.

These people are the reason I wanted to write this book. Infertility statistics are getting worse and our health as a general population is on the decline. Who knows what the fertility rates will be in 10 years' time. Keeping my knowledge to myself would help no one. So, I had to write this book.

My pivotal moment

I often think about what my pivotal moment was in my 10-year journey with infertility and recurrent miscarriage, the moment that sticks out in my mind the most. When I think back, it has to be the moment at age 41 when I had just miscarried my IVF baby at six weeks. In the review meeting with my fertility doctor afterwards, she said that my eggs were just too old and the only option from here was to go down the route of donor eggs. Prior to this moment, IVF was what we were always building up for. It was the last chance option to get pregnant if all else fails.

We started seeing a fertility doctor when we had been trying to conceive for about 12 months. Financially, we couldn't afford to do IVF straight away, so we went on the waiting list for publicly funded IVF treatment, and we had to wait 18 months for our chance to come up. We always knew that IVF was ahead of us and during that time we tried to be as healthy as we could be. In the back of our minds though, was the knowledge that we needed IVF, and it was likely to be the only chance we had of getting pregnant. We spent a lot of time building up to this moment.

After the initial round of tests, I was told I had low AMH, which was in the red danger zone for age 39. This suggested that I had a low ovarian reserve. It was a shock to us at the time as I wasn't over the age of 40 yet and we thought that we still had plenty of time.

Anti-Mullerian Hormone (AMH)

The AMH test, which stands for anti-mullerian hormone, is a routine blood test completed by fertility clinics to estimate ovarian reserve. It is usually completed prior to an IVF cycle as it helps to predict how many eggs you are likely to get in an IVF cycle. It can also help identify women who are at risk of early menopause and will therefore have reduced fertility earlier than average. According to Fertility Associates, a New Zealand-based fertility clinic, even though the test can help to pick up females who may lose their fertility more quickly, it cannot show who is more fertile than average. Nor can it predict ovarian reserve in people in PCOS.

Like most fertility tests, the AMR test does not give a black and white answer. Your score will either be in the green zone (above the 25th centile for young fertile women), orange zone (between the 25th and 10th centiles) and red zone (below the 10th centile).

Because my AMH was in the red zone at age 39, my doctor suggested that IVF was the best option for me. This meant that it was below the 10th centile for younger female women and predicted a 20% chance of six or more eggs in IVF.

This was pretty much spot on as when I had my only round of IVF at age 40, they retrieved five eggs. Out of the five eggs, three fertilised, which were great odds for my age. By the day five transfer, I had only one remaining embryo, as the other two did not survive. This meant I had no viable embryos to freeze.

The one egg that fertilised did well, and I ended up having a successful transfer, which despite the odds resulted in a pregnancy. Sadly, I suffered a miscarriage once again at six weeks.

At my post miscarriage review meeting with my fertility doctor, I was told that my eggs were too old and the only way forward from here was to use donor eggs. We decided we didn't want to do this and parted ways with our fertility clinic. At age 41, this felt like it was the end of the road.

Even though I should have just given up at this point, I had this gut feeling that I still needed to keep myself as healthy as I could, just in case. I was determined to be the healthiest version of myself I could possibly be.

I told those around me that I had stopped trying to conceive, but in reality, I was still hopeful. Those of you who have been on a fertility journey know it is hard to give up hope completely after such a long time. There is always a "what if?" in the back of your mind. It is only when something out of your control happens, like menopause, that you can finally admit it is over. I knew I would probably carry on hoping until I hit menopause.

All the hard work, stress, and tears paid off though as in June 2018, at age 43, I discovered with amazement that I was pregnant naturally. Despite all my previous losses, this pregnancy held on, and I gave birth to a healthy baby girl in February 2019 at age 44.

When I conceived, my health was the best it had been in my entire life. I had just spent three months on the GAPS gut healing protocol, so my digestive health was great with no bloating or discomfort. I also had unblemished skin, and I had gone nearly seven months without using an inhaler for my asthma, although my asthma came back when we got a kitten, but I didn't mind that as she made my son very happy.

So, if you are reading this and have also received the news that you have a less than favourable AMH score, just know that there is still hope. There are many things you can do to increase your chances and improve your egg quality. Don't just look to take a regime of dietary supplements, you will need to work on yourself and address any niggling symptoms that could contribute to a less than favourable environment for conception. I write about this in more detail in chapter 9 on silent inflammation. Even mild, easy to ignore symptoms can have an effect on you. Please know that the AMH test is just a predictor, and this can change. There is a reason to be hopeful and remember, it just takes one egg and one sperm.

Even after all my losses, I still had a gut feeling that I would have a baby in the end and that she was a girl, yes she was definitely a girl. It was weird that despite everything I remained calm and more determined than ever to do things my way.

This is why I wanted to write this book, as many couples believe IVF is their only option and they invest all their hopes into this one method. If it then fails, or they are told the donor route is their only option, they sadly give up trying. My story is proof that even when IVF fails and it seems like there is nowhere left to go, it is time to dig deep and go within to find answers. There is always hope, even if you feel like time is running out.

Why did it take me 10 years?

One thing you may wonder is why, if I am a practitioner specialising in fertility nutrition, did it take me 10 years to have a second child?

The truth is that a lot has changed over the last 10 years in terms of my journey, and how the natural health and nutrition industry has developed and evolved during this time.

When I first started trying to conceive a second child, it was 2009, and I had only just started studying nutritional science. So, when I had my first chemical pregnancy that year, I still had a lot to learn. As I moved through my studies and my knowledge of nutrition and the human body increased, I adapted my approach and experimented with many dietary and supplement protocols.

A lot of the important testing that I can organise for my clients now (such as a full thyroid panel, DUTCH hormone test, and MTHFR gene mutation test) only really became available in the three years or so before my daughter was born. If I had access to these tests sooner, it may not have taken me so long. I will discuss these tests in more detail throughout the book.

I always had a gut feeling that there was something up with my thyroid and tried to get it tested with my doctor on several occasions, but as they only ever ran the TSH (thyroid-stimulating hormone) test it was always inconclusive and "normal". So, I did what many desperate people do and experimented with taking different thyroid supplements. This was not the best decision as I found out that I have more of a tendency towards hyperthyroidism than hypothyroidism, although some symptoms can overlap. I found that taking these supplements to support my thyroid was not the best idea and gave me heart palpitations and anxiety. What I later learned through my studies is that focusing on supporting the adrenal glands first is important, rather than purely focusing on the thyroid. This is because prolonged stress and impaired adrenal function often down-regulates the function of the thyroid gland. This highlights the importance of testing the HPA (hypothalamus, pituitary and adrenal) axis and the full cascade of reproductive hormones with the DUTCH complete dried urine test. It is great that this test is now available to order through most naturopaths, nutritionists, and other natural health practitioners.

THE MTHFR gene mutation test has only really been available for the last few years, but it is proving to be an eye-opener as most of my clients experiencing recurrent miscarriages and chemical pregnancies have tested positive for one or two of the genetic mutations. This affects their ability to convert folic acid into methylfolate, the preferred active form. Even though I took 500 mcg of methylfolate daily, I still took a multivitamin with a little folic acid in it right up to a year before I conceived Jenah. I wonder if switching to the prenatal multivitamin with methylfolate and B vitamins was an important change for me, as it has been for several of my clients. They say you don't know what you don't know.

It is frustrating that it took me 10 years to conceive a second child, and I would not wish this emotionally draining infertility journey on anyone. I do like to believe, though, that my daughter was born at the time she was supposed to be. That this was the plan the universe had for me all along. I believe she was waiting for everything to be finally aligned for us before she showed up.

Chapter One

My story

I will touch on my story throughout this book as I talk about each concept and what I learnt during the 10 years I spent trying to conceive a second child. This chapter is my story as an overview to give you an idea of what I went through and to offer some inspiration if you are on a similar journey.

My journey with secondary infertility and recurrent pregnancy loss started in 2010 when my son was one and I was 34. After a month of trying to conceive again, I discovered my period was late. I felt like I might be pregnant again as I had some unusual symptoms. I remember going into the local pharmacy to get a pregnancy test and not feeling thrilled about it, as I felt it was too soon after giving birth to my son in late 2008. Three days after my positive pregnancy test, I started to bleed while having morning tea with my son. Although I didn't feel ready to have another baby, the loss completely devastated me and made me realise I wanted another baby after all. I was then on a mission to get pregnant as soon as I could.

I started work at a local health store not long after my son's first birthday and worked weekends. There was a lot of downtime between customers as at the weekends there were no orders, so I spent a lot of time researching infertility between customers. I was also studying nutritional science, so I used my practitioner resources to access research studies and specialist supplements to try.

Over the next two and a half years, I sadly had another seven early pregnancy losses between four and five weeks, the type where you get an early (sometimes faint) pregnancy test but then bleed a few days later. These early pregnancy losses, known as chemical pregnancies, are not considered established pregnancies until your doctor confirms it with an HCG (human chorionic gonadotropin) blood test. This means you really need to get tested at the doctors as soon as you find out. I could have probably done this if I had made an effort to. However, I started feeling really anxious whenever I suspected it was happening and tried to ignore it until at least a week after my period was due.

During my first year of trying to conceive, I felt that I possibly had postnatal depletion after the demands of pregnancy as well as breastfeeding my son for 14 months. My doctor arranged a blood test for me, and my iron was extremely low with a ferritin of 22 (the normal range is 20–200 ng/ML). Ferritin is a blood protein that contains iron so it can help doctors understand your iron stores. When my son was born, I endured a long and complicated labour that ended with me having a postpartum hemorrhage with a blood loss of approximately 800mls. I had no choice but to have a blood transfusion as my hemoglobin was dangerously low and I became weak with a very pale complexion that really shocked me when I looked in the mirror. After the blood transfusion, I took an iron supplement for about three months until I had another blood test to review my iron levels. I remember getting a call from my nurse at the time saying my iron was fine and that I could stop taking my iron supplement, so I did.

A year later, I asked for a copy of my medical history from my doctor and discovered that my ferritin was only 22 ng/mL when the nurse on the phone told me I could stop taking iron. This is borderline anemia, as the reference range is 20 -200 ng/mL, and the optimal range should be around 70 ng/mL.

I wish at the time I had the knowledge to ask my doctor to check my vitamin B12 levels while I was there, as I know this would have been low as well and a deficiency can cause infertility and recurrent pregnancy loss. It wasn't until later in my journey that I discovered the importance of having adequate levels of other methylation nutrients, such as folate, B12, B6, and choline. I will go into more about this later in the book.

After 12 months of trying to conceive without success, I was referred to Fertility Associates in Hamilton. After our initial meeting with the specialist, we felt positive that we would have another baby within the next year. The specialist put us on the waiting list for IVF and told us it would be about 18 months away so to keep trying in the meantime. The routine tests the clinic completed on both of us came back as normal. There was no sign that male factor infertility was an issue, as my partner's sperm analysis test came back with positive results. We were aware that he had a varicocele though, so he took extra precautions like not bathing in hot water or getting too hot while cycling.

In 2012, around two and a half years after I started trying again, I became pregnant after a holiday in Fiji (see what happens when you have no stress in your life and plenty of sunshine!). I was so surprised and incredibly anxious when the pregnancy got to five weeks and there was still no sign of bleeding, even though I felt sick with panic every time I went to the bathroom. Passing the five-week mark gave me hope this pregnancy would progress and I would have the baby I wanted so badly. I went to the doctor and had my HCG pregnancy blood test done at five weeks and they confirmed my pregnancy and that my HCG numbers were rising satisfactory. Human chorionic gonadotropin (HCG) is a hormone that is produced by the placenta when you are pregnant, so it is used to confirm a pregnancy.

At six and a half weeks, we had a dating scan to confirm that my dates were correct. I felt hopeful and a little anxious arriving at the appointment but sadly, the sonographer could not find a heartbeat during the ultrasound. She suggested we return in a week to check again, as it could be because it was too early. Over the course of the week between my scans, I suddenly felt different and knew it was over. I felt like someone had switched my hormones off and I no longer felt pregnant. Sure enough, the scan at seven and a half weeks confirmed there was no heartbeat and that it was a blighted ovum. This is where the body absorbs the embryo that has stopped developing, leaving an empty gestational sac. I was so sad and cried for the next week.

My body didn't miscarry naturally, so after one week I had a dilation and curettage (D & C), which is a surgical procedure to remove the fetal tissue from my uterus. Knowing I was carrying around my dead baby inside me for a week was such a horrible feeling.

It took a while to recover from the D & C as I had excessive bleeding caused by a large uterine fibroid that was located at the top of my uterus. Uterine fibroids can be common in women over the age of 35 and can play a part in implantation issues, so I often wondered whether it was the fibroid causing me to have these early miscarriages. Uterine fibroids are often linked to estrogen dominance and a deficiency of vitamin D, which I discovered later in my journey with recurrent pregnancy loss. I will discuss estrogen dominance further in chapter five.

For the next four years, I continued to have chemical pregnancies. I lost count in the end but would average about three per year. I believe over the course of 10 years I had about 17 very early pregnancy losses between four and five weeks. Despite this, I had technically experienced only one confirmed miscarriage with HCG blood tests on my medical records, so I still needed two more confirmed miscarriages before any further investigations could take place (as three are needed).

In 2016, at the age of 41, I had a round of publicly funded IVF after being on the waiting list for 18 months. Prior to having the procedure, I had my AMH tested to check on my egg reserve. The results unfortunately were not very hopeful, as my numbers were in the red. This meant I was running out of time, so this IVF was probably my last hope. The procedure was reasonably successful though with five eggs collected (which doesn't seem many but was apparently good for my age) and three of them fertilised, which is great odds. By the day five transfer, I had only one remaining embryo as the other two didn't survive, which meant I had no embryos to freeze.

Knowing this was likely to be my last chance, the 10 days wait from embryo transfer until the day I took the pregnancy test was unbearably stressful. I also had to insert uncomfortable progesterone pessaries twice a day, which was not pleasant. I kept myself distracted with work and meditated twice a day to stay calm and tried to visualise my growing baby inside my uterus, hoping this would make a positive difference.

I will never forget the day I had to go to hospital to take my pregnancy blood test, which was on the morning of the 10th day post transfer. I felt extremely anxious for the rest of the day, knowing that I would receive a phone call in the afternoon to confirm my results.

I still remember the phone call to this day. The words I heard from the fertility clinic were "congratulations, you are pregnant! your HCG levels are 92, which is great for this stage." They prescribed me progesterone pessaries to maintain progesterone levels and reduce the risk of miscarriage. Because of my advancing age and history of recurrent pregnancy loss, they also prescribed me baby aspirin to increase blood flow, which I was to take during pregnancy and stop at 35 weeks.

I hoped that this was finally my chance after over six years of trying to conceive. I believed that with the progesterone, baby aspirin, and specialist's supervision, everything would work out for us this time. I really felt that this was our time, and we would finally have another baby.

Unfortunately, I began bleeding just before six weeks, so it wasn't meant to be. I started having a miscarriage while I was at work by myself in a health shop. After making the discovery while taking a trip to the bathroom in my break, I had to clean myself up, put on a smile and go back out to the shop floor to continue serving customers. This was one of the hardest things I have ever had to do. I recently saw a similar scenario while watching the character of Mel on the TV show Virgin River. Mel was pregnant and had a miscarriage while she was working at the doctor's clinic. The town was in the middle of a crisis with fires raging through the town, so she had to clean herself up and just get on with it despite the heartbreak you could clearly see behind her eyes. This was exactly how I felt at the time it happened to me. Watching Virgin River brought this all back.

When I eventually arrived home that night after finishing a long eight-hour shift at the health shop, I found a *"Congratulations on your pregnancy"* pack waiting for me. I could not look at it. I felt devastated.

Two weeks later, I had an appointment at the fertility clinic. My doctor confirmed that my HCG levels declined after five weeks and showed me a graph with a downward arrow representing my hormones. She confirmed that my miscarriage was likely to be because of my age and my poor egg quality. The meeting felt like the end of the road for my journey with assisted reproduction, as my doctor confirmed that because of my age and AMH results, the only way forward was to use donor eggs.

We knew we were reluctant to go down the donor route and left the clinic that day feeling like it really was the end of the road.

It was not the end of the road

After a few weeks of healing and throwing myself into my new job, I felt a growing determination to prove my fertility doctors wrong, that this really wasn't the end of my fertility journey. I was determined to do whatever it took to improve my chances and work on my egg quality and overall health. My mission was to become the healthiest version of myself I could be.

Over the next three years, I literally turned myself inside out to try to work out what was happening to me. As a nutritionist and natural health practitioner, I had the benefit of having access to research articles, industry knowledge, and functional testing. I worked on my hormones, thyroid function, adrenal function, gut health, liver health, and stress management. I also started meditating, and writing weekly to the universe, explaining about the baby I always wanted and asking for signs of what action I needed to take next.

I kept my little project a secret. As far as friends and family were concerned, we had stopped trying after our IVF procedure ended in miscarriage. I even downplayed it to my partner, as I felt stupid being hopeful when we had been told there was no hope without a donor.

Over the next two years, I sadly had another three chemical pregnancies, one when I was on holiday in Thailand. I avoided drinking alcohol for most of the holiday just in case only to start bleeding on the plane home.

In 2018, at age 43, I quit my job working in a health shop to focus purely on building my business. As well as working 30 hours per week in the shop, I also ran my nutrition clinic part-time and was busy with my sons' after-school activities, so life was pretty frantic.

During those first few weeks off work, I rested and brainstormed my life and business goals. It was about three weeks later that I noticed my period was late and expecting the usual fate, I waited until five weeks before I took a pregnancy test because I was scared to take it earlier. I was so surprised to have such a strong positive that I immediately booked an appointment with my doctor for the HCG blood test. My doctor confirmed my pregnancy, and my HCG levels were doubling nicely. I should have been pleased, but after so much disappointment, I honestly felt numb, which is my body's usual defense mechanism to protect me from the inevitable outcome.

At eight weeks, I had a dating scan. As I arrived in the car park, I suddenly felt overwhelmed with anxiety that they would not find a heartbeat like last time. However, in the appointment I was so relieved and excited to hear a strong heartbeat, and the fetal growth was bang on eight weeks, so this was really happening.

Despite my ongoing anxiety, my 12- and 20-week scans were perfect, showing a low risk of congenital abnormalities, which the medical professionals deemed excellent considering my age. I was even brave enough to fly to England just after my 20-week scan. This was the point I started to believe my little baby would finally arrive.

My miracle daughter Jenah arrived in February 2019 by emergency cesarean at 39 weeks, weighing nine pounds one, which was a healthy size. I was 44 years old when she was born, and she was and still is absolutely perfect in every way. I am still amazed that my ageing body could produce such a miracle naturally, and other than baby aspirin, I didn't need any medications or artificial hormones.

I hope my story provides inspiration and encouragement to others who have tried unsuccessfully to have a baby for a long time without success. To go from no hope at age 41 to deliver a healthy baby girl at age 44 is such a blessing. I would have felt hopeful after reading a similar story when I was in the thick of my infertility journey, which is why I wrote this book.

I often wonder what I did differently to hold on to this pregnancy when my body rejected so many in the past. I believe the main reason was reducing my stress levels and workload, which helped to balance my hormones. Perhaps my eight years of handling till receipts in a retail environment may also have been connected. The chemical compound poly chlorinated biphenyls (PCBs) on receipts are detrimental to fertility. PCBs are known to be a serious environmental toxin that can interfere with hormones.

I continued to eat an optimal fertility diet throughout my infertility journey and worked to heal most of my skin issues and asthma (by healing my gut) so that nothing would stand in my way. So maybe my immune system was more balanced, who knows? Maybe my little girl was just waiting for the right time to show up, and at this point in my life, everything was finally in alignment. I genuinely believe this.

I have learned so much about infertility over the last 10 years that I feel motivated to help people in this area, especially as I understand how emotionally draining it can be to struggle with infertility. My area of focus is preconception nutrition and wellness for both females and males. This includes diet, lifestyle, environment, stress management, gut health, addressing hormone imbalances, and reducing toxicity. Please contact me if I can help you.

I hope my story has inspired you to keep searching for answers if you are currently having fertility challenges and feel you are running out of time. There is always hope.

To finish this chapter, here is a quote that always kept me going. I have this written on the first page of my diary each year.

"The moment you are ready to quit is usually the moment right before the miracle happens. Please do not give up,"
Author unknown

Chapter Two

Secondary infertility

Secondary infertility is the inability to become pregnant or to carry a pregnancy to term following a previous successful pregnancy. It is typically diagnosed after you have been trying to conceive for six months without success.

Surprisingly secondary infertility is almost as common as primary infertility and can affect around 11 – 13% of couples in the US according to various sources. Interestingly I found a study published in 2012 that concluded that in 2010: 1.9% of child-seeking women aged 20-44 experienced primary infertility and 10.5% experienced secondary infertility.[1] This is more of a global study rather than just focusing on America, but it is a reflection of what I am seeing in my clinic as the majority of my clients are seeking help with secondary infertility.

Fertility New Zealand recognise that there is a lack of mainstream recognition of secondary infertility and as a result there is a general lack of sympathy and understanding towards it.

Secondary infertility can be a frustrating journey, especially if you didn't have any problems conceiving your first child. You may wonder what has happened to you and whether the birth of your first child has broken you.

This was me. My first son was born in 2008 after a healthy problem free pregnancy. We conceived him fairly easily after five months of trying. His birth though, was not so easy. I will share a little about this later. Despite making the decision to try again in early 2009, when he was just over 12 months old, it took me nearly 10 years to finally welcome a second child. My beautiful baby girl was born in early 2019.

The guilt and the blame

Even though secondary infertility is as common as primary infertility, it is not perceived by society to be a major problem as you already have a child. We are often told that we should be grateful that we have one child, as many people in the world aren't even able to have one.

While I felt grateful and totally blessed to have a son, I also felt angry at myself for not being able to get pregnant. I blamed myself for being broken and felt guilty that I couldn't give my son a sibling to play with. He would often ask in his preschool and primary years, "why don't I have a brother or sister?" or "when will I be getting a brother or sister?" I felt so bad for him, especially when all of his friends one by one started getting their own brothers and sisters, and some even had a second sibling as well. My most heartbreaking moment was when I caught my son in his room praying for a little brother or sister.

I found it really tough attending playgroups when my son was young as the talk was all about babies and every single one of my friends had a second child. With secondary infertility, you face the pain and reminders daily as you cannot hide from or block out babies and pregnancy because of the life stage you are already in with your child. Soon I was the only one out of absolutely everyone I knew in my friendship circle who didn't have a second or third child.

What are the causes?

Your doctor will investigate the many causes of secondary infertility, but if they find no reason, they will label you as "unexplained". These are some of the common causes which are usually investigated by your doctor and fertility clinic:

Egg quality and quantity

Your age affects the quality and quantity of your egg supply, and many women are choosing to have children later in life. If you are over the age of 35, your chances of conceiving each cycle are naturally on the decline.

Structural issues

The structural causes could include scar tissue in your uterus or damage/blockage in your fallopian tubes. If your doctor suspects any of these issues, you will most likely have a scan at the hospital where they will filter a blue dye through your fallopian tubes to check for blockages.

Endometriosis

You may have always had some mild endometriosis which didn't affect your ability to have a first child, but it may have worsened over time and is a problem now. Endometriosis is common and is where uterine tissue grows outside the uterus in locations such as the ovaries, fallopian tubes, or other organs such as the bowel. Depending on the severity of the endometriosis, the inflammation and scar tissue can lead to issues with egg quality, ovulation, and implantation.

Fibroids

Uterine conditions such as fibroids may be present and are common in women over the age of 35. Researchers have established a connection between estrogen dominance and fibroids, which can occur in 70% of women by the time they are 50. For further information about fibroids, check out chapter five.

Caesarean section scar defect

Another cause of infertility is a caesarean section scar defect that affects only a small minority of women. You may not have heard of it as it is not that well known or routinely tested for, but a small group of experts are working hard to raise awareness of the complication. In New Zealand, Catherine Woulf, a mother and journalist, became passionate about raising awareness about the topic. She discovered through her own research that it was the cause of her own secondary infertility. In the references, you will find links to her articles that were featured in the New Zealand media in 2018.

A caesarean section defect is where a small pocket or pouch forms on the scar that is on the inside of the uterus. C-section scar defects are fairly common, but usually not problematic for women. Sometimes though the defect 'can act as a reservoir, retaining menstrual blood from each cycle and remaining constantly inflamed.' [2]

The connection with infertility is that the excess fluid buildup can potentially interfere with the implantation of the embryo. In addition, old blood can act as a toxin that can damage cells, including sperm, and can cause miscarriage.

A sign that you may have this issue is if you suffer from abnormal spotting and bleeding between periods, painful periods, and pain during intercourse. 'Clinical studies revealed that a caesarean section scar defect may lead to abnormal uterine bleeding, dysmenorrhea, pre or post menstrual spotting, heavy or prolonged menses, pelvic pain, and secondary infertility.' [3]

It is important to know that a c-section scar defect only affects a small minority of women and not to panic if you are trying to conceive a second child and you had a c-section with your first child. 'While it is fairly common to have a defect in a c-section scar, about one in three will cause abnormal bleeding or spotting and it is rare for this to cause infertility.' [4]

If you are wondering if this may be affecting you, raise this with your doctor and push for an ultrasound to check for signs of abnormal fluid in the uterus. If necessary, show them the articles in the references. According to the experts, a simple surgery may be required to resolve the issue and improve fertility chances.

Hormone imbalances

The common hormone imbalances that can affect secondary infertility are estrogen dominance, low progesterone, low or excess androgens, and issues with low or excess cortisol, the adrenal hormone. Your doctor may not identify these issues via the standard day 5 or 21 blood tests.

We are very fortunate these days to have the ability to investigate hormones on a deeper level with a dried urine test called the DUTCH test, which stands for Dried Urine Test for Comprehensive Hormones. The DUTCH test includes hormone metabolites, organic acids, and methylation and oxidative stress markers. It is especially useful for investigating adrenal function, estrogen and progesterone balance, androgen deficiency or excess, and whether the metabolism of hormones is sluggish or overactive. I can organise a DUTCH test for my clients, and I am trained to interpret the results, which can seem quite complex when you first look at them. The DUTCH test is a great way to investigate what is really happening with your hormones, as it not only provides information on free hormones but downstream metabolites as well, which tells us how the hormones are functioning. For further information, visit chapter five where I go into more detail about each of the common hormone imbalances.

Thyroid health

It is quite common to develop thyroid issues in the postpartum period after having your first child and for many, the changes in metabolism are permanent. This is called postpartum thyroiditis, and it can start a few months after birth and can last for several years afterwards. It can often be overlooked because the mother assumes her symptoms of low energy, hair loss and weight gain are just a part of being a new mum. I will go into more detail about this later in this chapter.

Autoimmune conditions

For many women, pregnancy can trigger the onset of one or more autoimmune conditions. Common examples of these are antiphospholipid syndrome, coeliac disease, psoriasis, lupus, Hashimoto's thyroiditis, Graves' disease, and rheumatoid arthritis. 'Research has shown that autoimmune diseases have a significant prevalence within the female population and a considerable portion of women who are mothers. 44.3% of women who develop an autoimmune disease have onset after the first year of pregnancy.' [5]

There are many theories why this occurs, such as fetal cells remaining in the mother postpartum and triggering an autoimmune response, as well as the stress and demands of pregnancy, hormone imbalances, and caesarean delivery, which increase the risk.

There are over 70 registered autoimmune conditions and many of these can go unnoticed and undiagnosed. With recurrent miscarriages, your doctor may test you for antinuclear antibodies (ANA) to see if you have elevated antibodies attacking your body tissues. They may also test for antiphospholipid antibodies (APA) to see if blood clotting is an issue as you may need to be prescribed low dose aspirin during pregnancy. Testing for coeliac disease (where gluten triggers an attack on the intestinal lining) and autoimmune thyroid disease, both Hashimoto's thyroiditis and Graves' disease are also important.

Ureaplasma

An infection of the urinary and reproductive tract called Ureaplasma may be problematic and can occasionally occur with severe cases of endometriosis and recurrent pregnancy loss. Ureaplasma is microscopic bacteria that can colonise in the urinary and reproductive tract and is usually harmless and asymptomatic for most women. An overgrowth of Ureaplasma can cause inflammation of the endometrial lining and may require a course of antibiotics to resolve. Ureaplama is not routinely tested for unless you are under the care of a fertility specialist or gynecologist. If you feel that Ureaplasma may also be an issue for you then it is worth pushing to get a test done.

Polycystic ovary syndrome (PCOS)

A common syndrome that can affect fertility is polycystic ovary syndrome (PCOS). Women with this syndrome may not ovulate and may have irregular periods. Females with PCOS may also have insulin resistance, high levels of androgens, excess hair growth, acne, and weight gain.

Lifestyle factors

Excessive weight gain in both males and females can also make it difficult to conceive, as well as smoking, alcohol consumption, excess sugar and refined carbohydrates. Also, the level and frequency of exercise can affect fertility as too much intense exercise is just as harmful as too little.

Male factor

In men, common reasons for infertility are a low sperm count, poor sperm motility, a varicocele, anti-sperm antibodies and other sperm abnormalities. These can be caused by environmental factors, inflammation, poor gut health and nutritional deficiencies.

Unexplained secondary infertility

Your fertility clinic may diagnose you as "unexplained" and recommend that you go on the waiting list for IVF if the standard blood tests and scans identify no obvious issue, just like in my case.

According to Fertility New Zealand, 15-25% of heterosexual couples receive a diagnosis of unexplained infertility. This is approximately one in five cases. Just because your fertility doctor has found no obvious reason why you can't conceive a second child, this is not the end of the road, because there is a whole world of further options to explore which may be outside the scope of practice for your doctor.

Postnatal depletion

I believe postnatal depletion is a major cause of unexplained secondary infertility. Mothers are so depleted of nutrients and energy from pregnancy and breastfeeding that they are just not physically capable of conceiving again until they build themselves back up.

Having a baby and breastfeeding is hugely demanding and can change a woman's body forever. During pregnancy and breastfeeding, the baby will strip all the nutrients it needs to grow from the mother's nutrient stores, leaving her at risk of nutritional deficiencies such as iron, calcium, vitamin B12, folate, and zinc. This nutrient depletion will affect the body's ability to function normally and, as a result, there can be subtle changes in metabolism and hormone health. In particular, the demands of motherhood and lack of sleep can cause the adrenal glands to become fatigued and dysfunctional, which can also affect the function of the thyroid and reduce progesterone levels. Many mothers may also be recovering from the emotional trauma of a difficult birth and maybe have (like I had) excessive blood loss, which can cause low iron and vitamin B12 that can take a while to return to healthy levels. So, when you try to get pregnant again in this state, your body is like NO WAY!

According to functional medicine doctor Oscar Serralach, author of the book *The Postnatal Depletion Cure*, postnatal depletion can affect mothers from birth until the child is seven years of age and possibly longer. Typical symptoms of postnatal depletion are fatigue, exhaustion, brain fog, hypervigilance, loss of self-esteem, overwhelm, and a loss of libido. [6]

I believe that postnatal depletion was an enormous factor with my secondary infertility journey.

My story

We conceived my first son fairly easily after five months of trying and my pregnancy was relatively straightforward with no major complications. I was 34 when he was born. Despite my problem-free pregnancy, my son's birth was far from easy. I won't go into all the details, but it was a long and painful labour lasting over 24 hours. He was a big baby, there were some complications, and they finally helped him out with an episiotomy and ventouse as he was stuck and unable to progress for a long time.

Immediately after I gave birth to my son, I had a massive postpartum hemorrhage, which required urgent medical attention, an experience that was very scary. I remember the doctor, nurses, and midwife all rushing around looking a little concerned, pressing on my stomach to get the placenta out and there was an awful lot of blood.

The day after, my health worsened, and the doctor informed me that a blood transfusion was necessary because my hemoglobin was critically low. Hemoglobin is the protein in your red blood cells that carries oxygen throughout your body. My hemoglobin level was about 92 g/L when it should be no lower than 114 g/L. The normal reference range for females is 120 g/L - 160 g/L. I didn't like the sound of a blood transfusion, however, after a chat with the doctor, I realised I would have no energy to look after my child unless I had one. So I reluctantly agreed to a blood transfusion.

My challenges didn't end there as I also had problems with my milk supply, and I wonder if the blood transfusion had caused this. After 10 days, my breast milk supply still hadn't come through, so I had to take a prescription drug to kick start my prolactin hormone production, which is the hormone that starts off the breastfeeding process. I also had to spend a lot of time expressing and topping up with formula milk, which was very stressful and meant that I spent little time sleeping.

Everything really took its toll in the first week after my son was born and, to make matters worse, I couldn't sleep! "Sleep when your baby sleeps" experts would say, but every time I tried to sleep, my mind was wide awake. I remember being so tired that I fell asleep while sitting up talking to the hospital canteen lady who took my food order. I literally didn't sleep for an entire week!

Looking back, I think about the huge emotional and physical toll of my son's labour and the weeks that followed, and how this affected my health. This is as well as the ongoing demands of 14 months of breastfeeding and seven months of my son waking multiple times during the night.

When my son was just over 12 months old, we decided to try for another baby. I didn't feel totally ready at first and hoped that it would take several months like last time. A few weeks later, I realised my period was late and so I took a pregnancy test at what would have been nearly five weeks. It shocked me to see it was a faint positive and I thought I would take another test the next day to make sure before saying anything to anyone, only to find that my period had arrived. This was likely my first chemical pregnancy.

Iron

Even though I wasn't ready to try again, experiencing an early pregnancy loss was very upsetting. It made me realise I wanted to get pregnant again after all, and I was determined to get pregnant again as soon as possible. As I had just started studying nutrition, I researched early pregnancy losses to try to understand why this might have happened to me. I also visited my doctor for further tests.

My doctor tested my iron levels as she was wondering if they were still low after my postpartum hemorrhage where I lost nearly 800 mls of blood. A couple of days after the blood test, I received a phone call from the nurse to say that my blood tests were normal, and no further action was required.

About three months later, I requested a copy of my blood test results and it surprised me to see that my "normal" ferritin was only 22 when the reference range was 20 -200 ng/mL.

Ferritin is a blood protein that contains iron and testing ferritin shows how much iron your body stores. I couldn't believe I was told my iron was normal when clearly it was just above the lowest reference range, showing my iron stores were very low. This would explain why I felt like a zombie most of the time. I knew I would be tired with the sleep deprivation of having a new baby, but I didn't have to feel so tired. Once I started taking iron, my energy levels improved gradually.

The impact of low iron on fertility

Iron deficiency anemia can be problematic if you are trying to conceive. It not only increases the risk of miscarriage, due to a lack of blood flow and oxygen to the uterus, but also plays an important part in a healthy thyroid function. This is because it is involved in the conversion of T4 (thyroxine, the inactive thyroid hormone) to T3 (triiodothyronine, the active thyroid hormone).

If your ferritin is very low, taking an iron supplement will not magically fix the problem, as iron can be slow to absorb and can take months to get your iron stores up to a healthy level. An optimal ferritin range is at least 70 ng/mL. This is why it is critically important to test iron levels as part of a three-month preconception care programme, especially for women who are looking to conceive a second child, as low iron could be a probability.

If your ferritin level is abnormally high but you still feel like your iron levels are low, it could be because of chronic inflammation or an infection, so it is important to consult with a practitioner to determine whether you need an iron supplement.

Eating liver a few times a week can help to increase iron levels, as liver is one of the richest sources of iron. Purchase a raw liver from your local butcher and keep it in the freezer. Grating liver into soups and stews that are being cooked on the stovetop is a good idea. This way, you won't even notice that you've added it. If you don't fancy eating liver, you can purchase grass fed liver capsules.

Zinc

Another mineral that is commonly deficient in mothers' postpartum is zinc, which, if not addressed, can have implications for future fertility. This is because zinc is an important mineral for reproductive hormone regulation, immune function and thyroid function as it is involved in the conversion of the inactive T4 to active T3. Zinc is antagonist to the mineral copper, so when one is elevated, the other can become deficient. Copper often becomes elevated during pregnancy and high copper levels postpartum can lead to zinc deficiency. This is one of the common patterns seen with postnatal depression and supplementing with zinc can be helpful. As well as postnatal depression, white spots on the fingernails, low appetite, and an altered sense of taste and smell are often signs of zinc deficiency.

Zinc is one of the key minerals depleted by stress as well, and the first few months postpartum are extremely stressful for the mother, both physically and emotionally.

As well as iron and zinc, vitamin B12, folate, vitamin D, and magnesium are also commonly depleted postpartum. It is important to work with a practitioner to get a comprehensive assessment of your vitamin and mineral status and a plan to replenish your nutrient levels with nourishing food and supplements. In the very least, a postnatal multivitamin and mineral supplement with activated B vitamins will help to boost nutrient intake.

Postpartum thyroiditis

During pregnancy, the thyroid gland works harder to produce around 50% more hormone than normal to support the baby's development.

Following pregnancy, many women experience postpartum thyroiditis, which often results in a fluctuation between hyperthyroidism (an overactive thyroid) during the initial three months and hypothyroidism (an underactive thyroid) between six to twelve months postpartum.

A common cause of postpartum thyroiditis is inflammation of the thyroid gland, which is often brought on by the physical changes of pregnancy and childbirth where the human chorionic gonadotropin (HCG) hormone stimulates the enlargement of the thyroid gland.

Dr. Sandra Cabot explains in her book *Your Thyroid Problems Solved* that postpartum thyroiditis has two phases. 'In the first phase, while the thyroid gland is inflamed, it releases too much hormone into the bloodstream. This phase usually lasts two to four months, and it causes the metabolism to speed up.' [7] Hyperthyroid symptoms are usually mild and often go unnoticed but typically would be symptoms such as weight loss, a rapid heart rate, anxiety, sleep issues, increased sweating, and a sensitivity to heat. It is easy to see how these symptoms may go unnoticed as many mothers' experience anxiety and sleep disturbances in the first few months postpartum.

In the second phase, the thyroid gland does not produce enough hormone, and this causes a swing to symptoms of hypothyroidism, which can last up to a year and sometimes longer. Typical symptoms can include goitre, which is a swelling of the thyroid gland, fatigue, depression, weight gain, hair loss, sensitivity to the cold, constipation, dry skin, and brittle nails.

Medical professionals consider postpartum thyroiditis to be an autoimmune disease because most women who develop the condition have elevated thyroid antibodies detected in their blood. According to Sandra Cabot, 'The body's immune system incorrectly identifies the thyroid gland as a foreign invader and produces antibodies to destroy it. While women are pregnant, their immune system becomes somewhat suppressed so that they don't produce antibodies that would harm the developing fetus. After delivery, the immune system becomes reactivated again, and it is during this time that the thyroid gland can become inflamed.'[8]

Women with pre-existing autoimmune conditions or a family history of autoimmunity have a higher risk of developing postpartum thyroiditis compared to those without.

I experienced the effects of postpartum thyroiditis for one to two years after giving birth to my son, but because of my limited knowledge of the thyroid at the time, I was unaware of the problem. I have coeliac disease, so I was a likely candidate to develop a further autoimmune condition after the huge amounts of stress my body physically went through with pregnancy and labour. In the first three months postpartum, I had increased symptoms of anxiety about my child, and I went through a phase of not being able to sleep as I was over vigilant about everything. My son woke a few times at night, but I found in those early months I would often struggle to fall asleep again. I would lie awake for hours, stressing about the fact that I couldn't get back to sleep during my small window of opportunity.

As the months went on, my symptoms changed to more hypothyroid symptoms such as fatigue, hair loss, dry skin, low body temperature, and an inability to lose weight. This was despite going to the gym and eating healthy. Unfortunately, my thyroid symptoms persisted for more than a year, making me one of the unlucky individuals whose symptoms didn't resolve within 12 months. When I started to try for a second child, I tracked my basal body temperature each day from day five to menstruation and was concerned that my temperature tracked around 35.5–35.8 C each day. The average basal body temperature for a healthy person is around 36.4–37.0 C. Both low thyroid function and low iron can cause metabolism to slow and body temperature to drop.

Testing

If you are concerned that you may have postpartum thyroiditis, then I recommend a full comprehensive thyroid panel to get an accurate picture of what is happening with your thyroid, although you may not be able to access this test via your doctor. A nutritionist, naturopath or functional medicine practitioner may be able to request this for you depending on their qualifications and scope of practice.

Whilst researching the thyroid, I came across this very important quote:

"Thyroid dysfunction can affect fertility in various ways, resulting in anovulatory cycles, luteal phase defect, high prolactin levels, and reproductive hormone imbalances. Therefore, normal thyroid function is necessary for fertility and to sustain a healthy pregnancy, even in the earliest days after conception. Thyroid evaluation should be done in any woman who wants to get pregnant with a family history of thyroid problems, irregular menstrual cycles, had over two miscarriages or is unable to conceive after one year of unprotected intercourse. The comprehensive thyroid evaluation should include T3, T4, thyroid stimulating hormone (TSH), and thyroid autoimmune testing such as thyroid peroxidase (TP0) antibodies, thyroglobulin/antithyroglobin antibodies and thyroid stimulating immunoglobulin (TSI)" [9]

In 2012, this study confirmed a need for a FULL investigation of the thyroid for anyone experiencing recurrent miscarriage or infertility issues. Yet here we are 10 years later and still most women experiencing infertility and recurrent miscarriage worldwide are not offered a full thyroid panel from their doctor, just TSH, and Free T4 if TSH comes back elevated.

During my 10-year journey with secondary infertility, I often had a gut feeling that I was having issues with my thyroid, although it was hard to prove as the limited tests that my doctor and fertility specialist were prepared to do at the time always came back within normal range.

This is a worldwide problem that affects many women, as conventional thyroid testing doesn't give a full picture of what is going on with the thyroid. As a result, many women live their lives with undetected thyroid issues, wondering why they rarely feel great.

As well as testing free T4, free T3 and reverse T3, the full thyroid panel test also includes the main thyroid antibodies, which is important to test to see if there is an autoimmune issue.

Additional support

I will go into more detail in chapter 8 on how you can naturally support your thyroid gland to function optimally. It is also important to support the hypothalamic pituitary adrenal (HPA) axis as part of a postpartum thyroid treatment plan. This is because it is often the stress of motherhood and the demands of breastfeeding and sleepless nights that takes its toll on the adrenal glands, which then down-regulates the thyroid gland. In chapter 7, I will go into more details on stress and adrenal function. It is also important to look at reducing potential immune triggers and supporting the immune system in postpartum thyroiditis, as it is considered to be an autoimmune condition driven by elevated thyroid antibodies. In chapter nine, I explore further how silent inflammation and autoimmunity may be a factor in unexplained infertility.

Chapter summary

Here are some actions you can take the implement the key points of this chapter:

- If you are considering trying for baby number two, it is important to spend at least three months getting your health back up to an optimal position for conception. Three months is the minimum time you want to be working on preconception care (the same for males as well) focusing on areas such as nutritional deficiencies, diet, gut health, hormones, thyroid, and adrenal health. It can take several months to recover from postnatal depletion, so if a second baby is on the cards, you will want to get started as soon as you can.

- It is important to get tested for iron, vitamin B12, folate, zinc and vitamin D, as it is common for these nutrients to be deficient postpartum.

- If you think you might have postpartum thyroiditis, consult with a practitioner to get a full thyroid panel completed to assess your thyroid function. While it's advisable to consult your doctor first and I encourage you to do so, most general practitioners typically only conduct TSH and Free T4 tests, which don't provide a comprehensive evaluation of your thyroid function.

Chapter Three

Building healthy foundations with nutrition

A s a nutritionist, I often get asked "what is the best diet for trying to conceive?" My answer to this question is that it really depends on the individual and their personal needs, goals, and preferences. We are all different and even with fertility, there is no ideal diet that suits everyone as our own genes, metabolism, and blood type can determine what foods are beneficial for us to eat. For example, some may need weight loss support, others gut health support or help with food intolerances, lowering inflammation or optimising a vegetarian diet. This is why most clients would benefit from a personalised diet plan.

There are, however, a few key principles of a fertility enhancing diet that you may wish to adopt if you are not already. These are:

Eat plenty of fruit and vegetables

Food is medicine, after all. Aim for around eight servings of fruit and vegetables a day if you are trying to conceive. Not just for the female, but for the male as well.

The optimal ratio is about six vegetables and two fruits a day with as much variety as possible. We need a rainbow of coloured fruits and vegetables a day to nourish the body with naturally occurring vitamins, minerals, and antioxidants. These nutrients are important to protect our cells from free radical damage, which includes the egg and sperm. Antioxidants are extremely important if you are trying to conceive over the age of 40 to combat age related oxidative damage.

As part of the six vegetables, have at least one serving a day of leafy green vegetables for natural folate. Great examples include kale, spinach, silver beet, rocket, mesclun, and broccoli. I will explain more about folate metabolism later in this chapter.

A variety of cooked and raw vegetables is important as well. If you have thyroid issues or feel the cold, then it would be beneficial to aim for about 70% cooked vegetables and 30% raw.

Achieving an intake of eight a day is easier said than done when you have a busy schedule. Here are some quick and easy ways to increase your fruit and vegetable intake:

Make a soup

In a food processor, blend meat stock with a variety of cooked vegetables such as pumpkin, carrot, celery, spinach, broccoli, and cauliflower.

Add to a smoothie

Use a variety of banana, berries, fruits, avocado, spinach, cucumber, and kale.

Raw juicing

The fruit and vegetables that work well for raw juicing include apple, pear, orange, mango, pineapple, carrot, beetroot, celery, cucumber, spinach, and kale.

Make a stir-fry

Use a variety of vegetables, such as carrot, celery, cabbage, broccoli, cauliflower, courgette, capsicum, and mushroom. You can add a protein such as fish, poultry, egg, meat, nuts, and seeds.

Make a frittata

A quick and easy dish with eggs and a variety of vegetables, such as pumpkin, spinach, broccoli, peas, carrots, capsicum, sweetcorn, and zucchini.

Make a salad

Salads are great in the warmer months using seasonal vegetables such as lettuce, tomato, cucumber, carrot, capsicum, radishes, spring onions, sprouts, beetroot, mesclun and baby spinach.

Steam or roast vegetables

A quick and easy dish is to steam some vegetables such as broccoli and cauliflower and top them with cheese.

Vegetable curry

Use a mix of vegetables like cauliflower, pumpkin, potato, peas, spinach, broccoli, and carrot to make a vegetable curry.

If you get to the end of the day and you have not quite had enough vegetables, there is always that jar of sauerkraut in the fridge. Instant vegetables at their finest.

Are you eating enough fat to conceive?

A diet low in healthy fats can be detrimental for fertility, as healthy fats are essential for manufacturing hormones. If you are eating a low-fat diet, you may not be ovulating as your body doesn't have the building blocks to make important reproductive hormones, such as progesterone.

I see this a lot in my clinic, as many of my female clients don't eat enough dietary fats. I think as a society we are still a little afraid of eating fat, after being conditioned with the "fat is bad" message for so long from public health agencies over the previous few decades.

The problem is fat is so critical for fertility and if you are not eating enough, you may not be ovulating. A lack of fat will also affect the function of all your cells, organs, and tissues, so it is not an ideal environment for conception.

If you are trying to conceive, I recommend having a good fat source with every meal (breakfast, lunch, and dinner). Some good choices are:

- Avocado

- Deep sea oily fish such as salmon, tuna, mackerel, and sardines

- Full-fat organic dairy products such as ghee, milk, butter, cheese, yogurt and kefir

- Coconut oil

- Olive oil

- Flaxseed oil

- Grass-fed meat

- Meat stock

- Nuts

- Seeds

Eggs

When trying to conceive, it is beneficial to eat eggs daily if possible. Eggs are a rich source of fertility boosting nutrients such as choline, B vitamins, vitamin A, omega-3 fatty acids, and protein.

If possible and affordable, choose organic and free-range eggs. Caged eggs may contain artificial hormones and antibiotics which may interfere with gut and hormone health. Luckily here in New Zealand our supermarkets no longer sell caged eggs.

Eggs support the adrenal glands

When we are under a lot of stress, our adrenal glands need extra support. Egg yolks are a building food and are rich in protein, cholesterol, vitamin A, zinc, and choline. Our adrenals and glandular system need fat and cholesterol to function and produce hormones, and egg yolks are the perfect food for this as they feed and nourish the glandular system.

If you are feeling exhausted and are experiencing adrenal issues, eating eggs daily can really help to rejuvenate your whole glandular system. This is why eggs are such an important food for fertility.

Choline

Choline is an essential nutrient for fertility and pregnancy that until recently was fairly overlooked. It is part of the vitamin B family. Research over the last 10 years has raised awareness of the role of choline as a methyl donor and how it is just as important as folate for lowering the risk of neural tube defects in babies. Choline is essential for fetal brain and nervous system development and improving cognitive function.

Eggs are the richest source of choline, so eating two eggs a day (preferably organic) can give you roughly 50% of your daily recommended intake of choline, which is 450 mg. Other sources of choline are meat, salmon, legumes, beans, and mushrooms.

Organic dairy products are the smarter choice for your hormones

Do you drink milk and eat cheese and other dairy products regularly? If you do, I encourage you to choose organic dairy products where possible and affordable for you.

This is because non-organic milk can contain a variety of added artificial hormones that act as endocrine disruptors. They play havoc with your hormones and can interfere with ovulation. If you regularly drink milk and are trying to get pregnant, choosing organic milk is a better option because it is free from hormones, antibiotics, and pesticides.

Raw milk is also beneficial for fertility as it is full of naturally occurring enzymes and vitamins which haven't been destroyed by the heat of processing. This helps us digest and absorb the nutrients from milk better.

Here are a few additional suggestions to optimise your fertility with nutrition:

- Avoid all empty calorie "beige" processed foods and refined sugar

- Eat nutritious whole foods made from scratch rather than processed foods

- Eat a good source of protein with most meals to support hormones and the growth and repair of body cells and tissues. Examples are meat, fish, poultry, legumes, nuts, and seeds

- Regularly consume fermented foods such as sauerkraut and kefir to support the health of your gut microbiome. I cover more on gut health later in the book

- Limit caffeine and alcohol

- Keep hydrated by drinking 30 mls of pure filtered water for each kg of body weight daily

My dietary approach

My dietary approach evolved over the 10 years I was trying to conceive my second child. This was influenced by my research as a nutritionist and my changing symptoms over the years.

As a coeliac, my main priority was being gluten free, but I later discovered the influential *Weston A. Price Foundation* dietary approach, especially in relation to fertility and pregnancy. I adopted their *Principles of Healthy Diets* for the last five years of my journey.

The Weston A. Price Foundation is a non-profit, tax-exempt charity founded in 1999 to disseminate the research of nutrition pioneer Dr. Weston Price whose studies of isolated non industrialised people established the parameters of human health and determined the optimum characteristics of human diets. The foundation is dedicated to restoring nutrient-dense foods to the diet through education, research, and activism. Central to Dr.

Price's research is the "fat soluble activators" vitamins found in the fats and organ meats of grass-fed animals, fish, eggs, and shellfish. Some of the key principles I adopted are:

- Opt for whole, unprocessed foods

- Include pasture-fed beef, lamb, organ meats, poultry, and eggs

- Consume wild fish and shellfish that are not farm-raised and come from clean, unpolluted water

- Choose full fat milk products from pasture-fed cows, favouring raw or fermented dairy

- Use animal fats such as lard, tallow, egg yolks, cream, and butter liberally

- Use only traditional vegetable oils such as extra virgin olive oil, flaxseed oil, and coconut oil

- Take cod liver oil regularly for vitamins A and D

- Eat fresh fruit and vegetables, preferably organic

- Prepare organic whole grains, legumes, and nuts by soaking or sprouting, to neutralise phytic acid, enzyme inhibitors, and other anti-nutrients

- Include enzyme-rich lacto-fermented vegetables, fruits, beverages, and condiments in your diet on a regular basis

- Prepare homemade stock from the bones of chicken, beef, lamb, and fish fed non-GMO feed and use liberally in soups, stews, gravies, and sauces

- Use filtered water for cooking and drinking

- Use unrefined salt and a variety of herbs and spices for flavour

- Consume traditional sweeteners like raw honey, maple syrup, and stevia in moderation

The Weston A Price dietary approach helped me to increase my intake of fat and protein after I realised I wasn't having optimal levels. According to research from Weston A Price, traditional diets provide at least TEN times more fat-soluble vitamins from animal foods such as butter, fish, eggs, shellfish, organ meats, and animal fats. My goal was to have a good source of fat with each meal, and butter became my new best friend.

Important nutrients for fertility

When you are looking to optimise your health to prepare for pregnancy, it is important to ensure you are eating optimal levels of the key nutrients for fertility. Doctors and fertility specialists often overlook nutritional deficiencies when conducting review appointments, but they are an important part of the overall picture.

Here are some important vitamins and minerals to optimise when trying to conceive.

Iron

Iron is one of the most important minerals to investigate in cases of infertility and recurrent miscarriage, but also for general preconception care and pregnancy.

During pregnancy, the volume of circulating blood in the body increases by approximately 40%, which is a very demanding time for the mother. We need adequate iron stores for the increased production of haemoglobin; the oxygen-carrying component of the blood.

When blood does not get enough iron, there is an insufficient number of red blood cells and anaemia can develop. If someone suffers from anaemia, they lack enough healthy red blood cells to carry adequate oxygen to all body tissues and organs, including the uterus. This can cause a poor oxygen supply to the fetus, which can lead to pregnancy complications and even miscarriage.

Iron also supports the immune system of the mother and is involved in thyroid hormone conversion in the liver (T4 to T3). Sufficient iron is essential for the development of fetal blood, as well as the baby's brain, eyes, and bones.

For fertility, a reduced supply of oxygen to the ovaries and uterus may cause poor egg quality, anovulation (lack of ovulation), and reduced chances of conception. If conception occurs, anaemia makes it difficult for the cells of the growing fetus to divide and grow properly, which can increase the risk of miscarriage.

Those at risk of iron deficiency are:

- Vegans and vegetarians as red meat is the most absorbable source of iron

- Inflammatory gut disorders, as inflammation in the gut inhibits the absorption of minerals. These are conditions such as IBS, coeliac, and Crohn's disease

- Females with heavy periods

- Females who exercise excessively

Typical symptoms of iron deficiency:

- Mild to severe fatigue

- Chronic headaches, dizziness

- Shortness of breath, palpitations

- Brittle or weak nails with longitudinal ridges

- Restless legs

- Decreased appetite

- Low blood pressure

- Cold hands and feet

- Pale skin, nails and tongue

- Nails spoon shaped or separating from the nail bed

- Craving non-food items such as paper or dirt

Iron-rich foods to include in your diet are beef, lamb, pork, liver, chicken, beetroot, leafy greens such as spinach and kale, beans, lentils, tofu, avocado, molasses and dried fruit.

Beef and lamb are haem sources of iron and have a higher absorption rate than non haem plant sources of iron.

Eating foods high in vitamin C alongside iron-rich foods helps with the absorption of the iron. Good examples of foods rich in vitamin C are citrus fruits, strawberries, broccoli, capsicum, and potato.

If you are low in iron and you need to take a supplement, my favourite form is iron bisglycinate which is a well-absorbed type of iron that isn't affected by calcium-rich foods and grains which can reduce the absorption of other types of iron. If you are low in iron, it can take a little while to get your iron up to healthy levels, so I recommend you get your iron levels checked before you try to get pregnant.

Adding grated raw liver from the freezer to soups and dishes cooking on the stove can be a great way to increase iron levels, as liver is one of the richest sources. If you dislike the taste of liver, consider beef liver capsules as a substitute.

Iodine

The trace mineral iodine is important for fertility and is required daily in small amounts. It is essential for a healthy metabolic rate, the function of a healthy thyroid gland, and the prevention of goitre, which is the abnormal swelling of the thyroid gland.

To make thyroid hormone, the body uses molecules of iodine and the amino acid tyrosine, which you can get by eating protein-rich foods such as organic animal meats, poultry, eggs, fish, nuts, seeds and dairy products.

Iodine is important during the preconception period and throughout pregnancy for the growth and development of a healthy baby. It is important for the development of the baby's central nervous system. Low levels of thyroid hormone can cause women to stop ovulating, leading to infertility.

In New Zealand, iodine is very deficient (even absent) in our soils. People rarely eat foods that are rich in iodine such as seaweed, kelp, and saltwater fish, which compounds the problem. We have been misled into believing that all salt is bad for our health (which is not true unless we have severe hypertension), so many people are avoiding salt, even though it is an excellent source of iodine. Rather than avoid salt completely, make sure you are getting some healthy salt in your diet, such as Himalayan pink rock salt or Celtic Sea salt, which are rich in naturally occurring minerals, including iodine.

Some key signs that you might have iodine deficiency:

- Underactive thyroid gland

- Goitre

- Low body temperature

- An oversensitivity to the cold

- Fatigue and weakness

- Inability to lose weight and gains weight easily

- High HDL cholesterol

- Infertility and recurrent miscarriage

- Fibrocystic breasts and painful breast lumps

- Dry skin or mouth

- Hair loss, outer third of eyebrow missing

- Constipation

- Cancer of the breast, prostate, ovaries, thyroid, or uterus

The recommended daily dosage for iodine supplementation is 150 mcg per day of potassium iodide however this may not be enough if you are severely deficient in iodine. In addition, you must be careful not to take too much iodine (over 600 mcg daily) as excess iodine intake may inhibit the secretion of thyroid hormone further and make your hypothyroidism symptoms worse. It may also tip you over into a hyperthyroid state or cause a thyroid storm or thyrotoxic crisis (an excessive release of thyroid hormone) which can be dangerous. If you develop a high fever and rapid heart rate this could be a thyroid storm so a trip to hospital to get checked out is advisable. Please note that iodine supplementation is not recommended and can be harmful if you have an overactive thyroid (hyperthyroidism) so if you are concerned it is best to consult a healthcare practitioner before taking iodine supplements. It is also advisable to be cautious with excess iodine if you have Hashimoto's thyroiditis as iodine can make symptoms worse in some people.

Good food sources of iodine are seaweeds such as kelp and bladderwrack, iodized salt, sea salt, eggs, seafood, saltwater fish, and dairy products. Sprinkling kelp powder on your meals is a great way to get a daily dose of iodine.

Raw brassica foods such as broccoli, kale, cabbage, Brussels sprouts, and cauliflower are goitrogenic foods that block the uptake and absorption of iodine so if you have (or suspect) you have a thyroid problem, it is best to not have too much of these vegetables raw. Cooking inactivates the goitrogens so lightly steaming or stir-frying brassica vegetables is acceptable. Many people add raw kale to their juices daily, believing they are being healthy without realising that it can be problematic to your thyroid health. Excess soy consumption can also interfere with iodine absorption, but moderate soy consumption does not impact on thyroid health.

Fluoride, chlorine, and bromide are chemicals found in our environment that bind to iodine receptors in the thyroid and block the absorption of iodine. Some ways we can protect our thyroid:

- Use a natural fluoride-free toothpaste

- Filter all drinking water

- Use a shower filter so you do not inhale chemicals from the water

- Avoid non-stick frying pans as they contain fluoride and bromide that are released when heated

- Buy organic fruits and vegetables where possible

Zinc

Zinc is an important mineral for reproductive health as it is involved in over 300 enzyme functions in the body. Without adequate levels of zinc, cells cannot divide properly, which is why it is so important for egg and sperm health. In terms of the fetus, zinc plays a role in brain formation, immune function and skeletal system development.

Both the male and female reproductive systems can't function efficiently without zinc. A deficiency can contribute to low thyroid function, hormone imbalances and can increase the risk of miscarriage.

We need zinc for several key reproductive functions, these include:

Egg production

Females need adequate zinc to produce mature eggs that are optimal for fertilization.

Follicular fluid levels

Zinc helps to maintain follicular fluid levels. Without enough fluid in the follicles, an egg cannot adequately travel through the fallopian tube and into the uterus for implantation.

Hormone regulation

Zinc plays a crucial role in regulating estrogen, progesterone, and testosterone levels throughout the menstrual cycle and is important for thyroid function.

Male fertility

Optimal zinc levels are essential for male fertility as zinc can increase sperm count and improve the form, function, and quality of sperm.

If you are supplementing with zinc, it is advisable to take it away from any supplements that contain calcium, iron, and copper, as they can deplete zinc. The contraceptive pill also depletes zinc, so checking your levels during the preconception period is important.

Common zinc deficiency signs:

- Weak immune system

- Poor memory

- Loss of taste and smell

- Sleep problems, as we need zinc to make melatonin

- Hair loss

- Loss of appetite

- Low libido

- Slow wound healing

- White spots on fingernails

- Pale nails

- Low thyroid function

- Infertility

- Hormone imbalances, such as low testosterone or progesterone

Good food sources of zinc are liver, oysters (although avoid if you become pregnant), beef, lamb, venison, eggs, sesame seeds, pumpkin seeds, yogurt, green peas, mushrooms, tahini, and dark chocolate.

Selenium

Selenium is an antioxidant mineral that helps to protect cells from free radical damage. There are low levels of selenium in New Zealand soils so many people are deficient if they are not eating enough selenium rich foods.

Selenium helps to modulate the immune system and regulate thyroid function as it is involved in the conversion of T4 to T3 in the liver. It may also help to protect against birth defects and miscarriage. As a powerful antioxidant, selenium is important for egg production.

Having adequate selenium in your diet is important if you have an autoimmune condition such as Hashimoto's thyroiditis, coeliac disease, Crohn's disease, lupus, and psoriasis as it modulates and calms down an excessive immune response.

If you are over the age of 40 and trying to conceive, selenium may help to reduce the risk of having a child with congenital abnormalities.

Men require selenium for the creation of sperm, and a deficiency in selenium is associated with low sperm count and motility.

Common deficiency signs:

- Hair loss

- Discolouration of nails and skin

- Tiredness

- Brain fog

- Hypothyroidism

- Infertility

- Poor immunity

- Autoimmune diseases

One of the easiest ways to get selenium in your diet is to eat three Brazil nuts per day as they contain an average of 68 -91 mcg per nut. Other food sources are tuna, sardines, grass-fed beef, liver, chicken, egg, and spinach.

The recommended dietary intake (RDA) for selenium is 150 mcg in total from all supplements. This is because of the risk of toxicity with very high amounts over 200 mcg daily. So, check that you are not getting too much from other sources like your multivitamin. A qualified practitioner may recommend a higher dose if you have an autoimmune condition, however this is dependent on the individual.

Omega 3

Omega-3 essential fatty acids (EFAs) are very important for fertility and pregnancy. We consider them essential because the body cannot manufacture the important forms of omega-3 ourselves, which include eicosapentaenoic acid (EPA), docosahexaenoic acid (DHA), and alpha-linolenic acid (ALA). It is therefore important to supply these through your diet.

Fatty fish such as salmon, tuna, mackerel, and anchovies are good sources of EPA and DHA. Walnuts, chia seeds, hemp seeds, flaxseeds, flaxseed oil, and hempseed oil contain ALA.

Omega-3 essential fatty acids are beneficial for fertility by helping to regulate hormones, increase cervical mucus, promote ovulation, and increase blood flow to the reproductive organs. Omega-3 is also important for the structure of ovarian cell membranes.

DHA is an essential fatty acid for brain health. Research has linked low levels of DHA to depression and other mental health issues. It is also important for the development and function of the brain and nervous system of the baby.

Many females with unexplained infertility have low-grade chronic inflammation, which has a negative effect on egg quality. Issues such as poor gut health, food intolerances, infections, and exposure to toxins can cause inflammation.

Omega-3 is one of nature's most important anti-inflammatories, which, when consumed regularly in food and supplement form, can help to reduce unhealthy levels of inflammation.

How omega-3 essential fatty acids promote fertility:

- Helps to regulate hormones and promote ovulation

- Increases blood flow to the uterus

- Improves embryo quality

- Increases egg white cervical mucus

- Reduces inflammation

What about our men? Here are some of the major benefits for male fertility:

- Omega-3 essential fatty acids improve circulation to the genitals, which helps to support the prostate and reproductive organs

- Sperm cell membranes are rich in omega-3, which helps to support the flexibility and motility of sperm cells.

- Supports healthy sperm production

Common omega-3 deficiency signs are:

- Dry skin

- Dry eyes

- Hangnails on the side of the nails

- Brittle nails

- Skin rashes, eczema

- Memory and concentration issues

- Anxiety, mood issues

- Inflammation, joint pain

It is advisable that pregnant women limit their fish intake to around three times a week to avoid the potential risk of mercury exposure, and supplement with a good quality prenatal DHA fish oil, such as the Nordic Naturals brand. It is best to start taking omega-3 at least three months before trying to conceive for optimal results.

Cod liver oil

One of the key supplements I recommend for my fertility clients is cod liver oil, a traditional food that is very beneficial for both male and female fertility. It should ideally be taken for at least three months prior to conception and women would also benefit from taking it during pregnancy and lactation.

Cod liver oil is an excellent source of vitamins A and D and EPA and DHA, which, as we know, are essential for the development of the brain and nervous system. It can also help to reduce inflammation in the body.

Vitamin A benefits

Vitamin A, found in cod liver oil, is essential for the development of the oocyte, the ability of the egg to implant, and the growth and development of the embryo. A lack of vitamin A can reduce luteinising hormone (LH), which is important for ovulation. Vitamin A is also important for thyroid health.

Vitamin D benefits

Researchers have linked vitamin D (a hormone-like substance rather than a nutrient) as such, to fertility problems. It helps to regulate the immune system and is important for calcium absorption and bone health. Vitamin D also helps the body to manufacture reproductive hormones, such as progesterone and estrogen, and support thyroid problems.

Saturated fats such as butter can help transfer DHA into our tissues, allowing it to work more effectively. So, it is a good idea to take your cod liver oil when you eat butter.

Nutrition pioneer Western A Price considered the fat-soluble vitamins (especially vitamin A), to be the "catalysts on which all other biological processes depend." Efficient mineral uptake and utilisation of water-soluble vitamins require sufficient Vitamin A in the diet. His research showed that adequate amounts of vitamin A promotes healthy reproduction and healthy babies.

Taking a teaspoon a day of cod liver oil, or fermented cod liver oil, will provide sufficient vitamin A at safe levels. It is important not to exceed the upper limit of 10,000 iu per day.

According to Sally Fallon, author of *Nourishing Traditions*, Regular cod liver oil contains 5,000 iu per teaspoon and fermented cod liver oil about 5,000 iu per half a teaspoon.

Vitamin B6

As a hormone regulator, vitamin B6 plays a substantial role in reproductive health. Supplementing with vitamin B6 can be helpful if you have a luteal phase defect, which is a shorter luteal phase of 10 days or less. Vitamin B6 helps to increase progesterone levels and adequate progesterone levels are necessary for preparing the endometrium for implantation. Vitamin B6 also inhibits the excess production of prolactin, which may be caused by a dysfunctional pituitary gland.

As a methyl donor, adequate vitamin B6 levels are also important for liver detoxification, the clearance of excess hormones via the liver, and regulating homocysteine levels. High homocysteine levels are linked to infertility and recurrent pregnancy loss. Vitamin B6 is also a key nutrient for energy metabolism and mental health. For men, vitamin B6 is important for sperm health and motility.

Common B6 deficiency signs:

- Irritability

- Anxiety

- Depression

- PMS symptoms

- Breast tenderness

- Muscle pains

- Low energy

- Fatigue

- Fluid retention

Good food sources are tuna, pork, eggs, banana, liver, salmon, spinach, capsicum, garlic, cauliflower, celery, cabbage, broccoli, kale, and wholegrain cereals.

To ensure you are getting adequate vitamin B6, I would take a prenatal multivitamin with at least 50 mg of activated B6, as pyridoxal 5 phosphate (P5P). Vitamin B6 as pyridoxine, which is the standard form in most supplements, must be converted by the liver to P5P for it to be effective. Some people with autoimmune and inflammatory conditions may have trouble converting pyridoxine to the active form of P5P, so taking P5P as a supplement is better utilised by the body.

Vitamin C

Vitamin C is a superstar nutrient that has multiple functions in the body. It is important for a robust immune system, the production of adrenal hormones, the metabolism of essential fatty acids, and the absorption of iron.

A diet rich in vitamin C can protect against genetic abnormalities in both the sperm and the egg. Vitamin C is abundant in the ovaries, emphasizing its role in follicle growth, ovulation, and corpus luteum development. Supplementing with vitamin C after ovulation may lengthen the luteal phase and improve progesterone levels.

In men, studies have shown that vitamin C improves sperm quality, protects sperm from DNA damage, and prevents sperm from clumping together, making them more motile.

Stress, smoking, and infections can reduce levels of vitamin C. When you are stressed, consume plenty of vitamin C rich foods to support your adrenal glands. This is because vitamin C gets depleted more rapidly during periods of stress and the adrenal glands depend on vitamin C to produce important adrenal hormones.

Vitamin C deficiency signs:

- Poor immunity

- Poor wound healing

- Rough skin

- Bleeding gums

- Easy bruising

- Fatigue

- Dandruff

Foods that are rich in vitamin C are red peppers, broccoli, citrus fruits, strawberries, kiwifruit, tomatoes, spinach, cabbages, and potatoes.

If you choose to supplement with vitamin C, I recommend the liposomal form for advanced absorption.

Vitamin D

Vitamin D can often be the missing link in cases of infertility. It is such an important vitamin because it is a cofactor for around 2,000 genes in the body.

Our skin produces vitamin D3 (cholecalciferol) when exposed to the sun, which is why it is known as the sunshine vitamin. If we spend enough time out in the sun on a daily basis, most of us could make enough vitamin D. However, many of us do not get enough consistent sun exposure to maintain normal vitamin D levels throughout the year, with levels dropping over the wintertime.

Foods such as eggs, cod liver oil, mushrooms, fatty fish (such as tuna and salmon), and cow's milk also contain vitamin D3, but it is difficult to get enough through the diet.

A deficiency in vitamin D3 has been associated with various autoimmune conditions, as it has a regulatory effect on the immune system. As many fertility issues can result from an underlying autoimmune condition, it is important to get your vitamin D levels checked.

In terms of IVF, taking vitamin D has been shown in studies to have a positive impact on IVF outcomes. [1]

According to a 2014 study, vitamin D3 modulates reproductive processes in both men and women. The study concluded that 'in women undergoing in-vitro fertilization, a sufficient vitamin D level (> 30 ng/ml) should be obtained as this is associated with higher pregnancy rates. Vitamin D supplementation might improve metabolic parameters in

women with PCOS. A high vitamin D intake might be protective against endometriosis.'
2

In men, vitamin D is essential for the development of healthy sperm and improved sperm count. It also helps to support healthy testosterone levels.

Vitamin D deficiency signs:

- Infertility

- Excess sweating

- Muscle weakness

- Chronic infections

- Weak bones, bone pain

- Chronic pain

- Tiredness

- Depression (as it affects levels of serotonin in the brain)

- Digestive issues

- Asthma

To enable your skin to make vitamin D, try to spend 15 minutes every day out in the sunshine with no sunscreen on throughout the year. In summer, it is best to avoid the heat of the day so before 10.00 am and after 3.00 pm is the best time. Your skin will manufacture vitamin D when it is in contact with the sun. In the winter, you need to be in the sun for at least one hour to manufacture enough vitamin D.

If you are trying to conceive as a minimum, it is recommended to take 2,000 IU of vitamin D3 per day, possibly more depending on your test results. It is important to have your vitamin D levels monitored regularly to ensure you are taking adequate amounts.

Folate

Vitamin B9, otherwise known as folate, is one of the most important nutrients for fertility and pregnancy. We need folate for the development of red blood cells and DNA. As folate plays a crucial role in cell division, it is crucial for both egg and sperm health.

Folate helps to prevent neural tube defects, congenital heart defects, cleft lip, limb defects, and other abnormalities in the developing fetus.

A deficiency in folate increases the risk of premature babies, low birth weight and an increased risk in miscarriage due to high homocysteine levels in the blood. Folate helps to support ovulation and progesterone levels, and is important for methylation, an important phase two liver detoxification pathway.

Typical folate deficiency signs:

- Fatigue

- Anemia

- High homocysteine levels

- Weak immune function

- Poor digestion

- Canker sores in the mouth

- Tender swollen tongue

- Geographic tongue, which is patches of clear tissue like a map

- Low mood

- Pale skin

- Premature grey hair

Long-term use of the contraceptive pill depletes folate levels, and it can take up to three months to re-establish levels after stopping the pill. This highlights the importance of at least a three-month preconception care plan before trying to conceive.

Leafy green vegetables are the best source of natural folate and are easy to include in your diet daily. Examples are kale, spinach, broccoli, silver beet, Brussels sprouts, mesclun, romaine lettuce, mustard greens, and rocket. Other food sources are lentils, liver, rice, asparagus, avocado, sweetcorn, and oranges.

As a general rule, it is best to supplement with at least 800 mcg of folate per day, preferably as calcium l-5-methyltetrahydrofolate (5-MTHFR) instead of folic acid. Depending on your age and previous medical history, you may need a higher dose, especially if you are over the age of 40.

Folate is the active form of vitamin B9 that is well absorbed in the small intestines. Folic acid, on the other hand, is a man-made synthetic version that needs to undergo various steps in the liver to convert to 5-methyltetrahydrofolate. Many people have problems converting folic acid to the active form of folate in the body, which is why it is important to supplement with folate and eat plenty of foods rich in folate such as a daily serving of leafy greens. Let's go into this in more detail.

Why you should avoid ALL sources of folic acid in favour of methylfolate

Over the last seven years there has been a lot of emerging research available about the negative effects of folic acid and how if you are trying to get pregnant, supplementing with active folate (methylfolate) is the preferred choice. This is because of a MTHFR gene mutation that affects approximately 50% of the population.

What is the MTHFR gene mutation?

The MTHFR gene is one of around 20,000 genes in the human body. It provides instructions that regulate the production of methylenetetrahydrofolate reductase, which is the MTHFR enzyme that converts folic acid into methylfolate in the methylation cycle. Around 50% of the population has a genetic mutation or SNP that occurs in the MTHFR gene, which is a slight variation in the DNA sequence.

A MTHFR gene mutation blood test can identify the two common MTHFR genes, which are C677T and A1298C. The test can identify if you have no mutations, one mutation (heterozygous), or two mutations (homozygous) on either or both of the genes. The more mutations you have, the lower the MTHFR enzyme activity and, therefore, a reduced conversion into methylfolate. It reflects decreased methylation and detoxification function.

If you have a mutation in your MTHFR gene, your body cannot convert synthetic folic acid into its active form 5-methylenetetrahydrofolate (5-MTHFR) via the methylation cycle. What this means is there is less active folate available even if you are taking high doses of folic acid. It also means that the large doses of folic acid end up as unmetabolized folic acid in the bloodstream, which can block the methylation cycle and can contribute to many chronic health conditions.

Yet despite this information being widely available, there are still some fertility clinics supplementing their clients with a whopping 5 mg daily dose of folic acid. Why is this message not getting through? According to a study published in the *Journal of Assisted Reproduction and Genetics in* 2018 'The conventional use of large doses of folic acid (5mg/day) has become obsolete. Regular doses of folic acid (100-200 mg) can be tolerated in the general population but should be abandoned in the presence of MTHFR muta- tions, as the biochemical/genetic background of the patient precludes a correct supply of 5-MTHF, the active compound.' [3]

It can be quite complex and confusing to understand all this, so I will try to explain it as simply as I can. It is so important that you are aware of this, as it could be affecting you.

What is folic acid and why is it detrimental for fertility for some people?

Folic acid is a synthetic man-made form of vitamin B9 that is not found in nature. It must undergo various conversion steps in the methylation cycle to become active folate (known as methylfolate or 5-MTHFR) a form that is utilised by the body and is important for healthy DNA.

Methylation is a simple biochemical process that involves the transfer of a methyl group (one carbon atom and three hydrogen atoms) from one substance to another. The most important methyl groups used in methylation are methylfolate (5-MTHFR), methylcobalamin (active B12), pyridoxal 5 phosphate (active B6), and choline. The issue is, if you have the MTHFR gene mutation (which roughly 50% of the population has) then the conversion to folate is disrupted. This is because the MTHFR enzyme (methylenetetrahydrofolate reductase) affects the last step of the methylation cycle, and the activity of this enzyme can be reduced by as much as 60% with a homozygous mutation.

If you eat foods rich in natural folate such as leafy green vegetables, it is already in the form of methylfolate. However, if you eat foods fortified with synthetic man-made folic acid such as bread and cereals, then your body must first convert the folic acid through all the steps down the methylation pathway until it gets to methylfolate (5-MTHFR). This means that despite eating plenty of folic acid (and even taking supplemental folic acid) your body remains deficient in folate if you have the MTHFR gene mutation.

The problem is that even a little folic acid from food can disrupt the methylation cycle, which is why the fortification of flour with folic acid could be problematic for some people. It is important to avoid all forms of folic acid from fortified foods and supplements and only take methylfolate (5-MTHFR) and eat folate rich foods like leafy green vegetables every day.

According to Dr Ben Lynch 'Because folic acid resembles folate, it gets into your folate receptors, where it blocks natural folate from getting where it needs to, inside your cell. As a result, if you are eating more foods containing folic acid than leafy green vegetables, the naturally occurring methylfolate struggles to get into your cells. And without enough methylfolate, your body can't methylate. In this way, folic acid blocks methylation.' [4]

As Folate is one of the most important nutrients for fertility, being deficient can affect your ability to conceive and increase your chances of pregnancy complications and recurrent miscarriage.

My story

It was about four years into my 10-year infertility journey that I first found out about the MTHFR gene, and I often wonder whether taking folic acid for the first few years had a negative impact on me. It was Dr. Ben Lynch who introduced me to the concept of MTHFR when I listened to one of his podcasts. The science was very new and confusing and even though I started taking active folate rather than folic acid, I still took a prenatal multi that had 400 mcg of folic acid in it out of ignorance. At the time, there were no prenatal multivitamins with activated folate on the market because the research was still very new. This has changed now thankfully as there are many prenatal multivitamins available with activated B vitamins now, such as Naturobest.

It was a few years later that I finally eliminated all folic acid from foods and supplements and a few months later I found out I was pregnant at the age of 43 after 10 years of secondary infertility. It wasn't the only change I made, but I believe cutting out folic acid made a difference.

I never got around to getting myself tested for the MTHFR gene, mainly because it was a new science on the scene and while I was trying to conceive, the only testing was expensive genetic testing from places like 23andme. You can now easily get a MTHFR gene mutation test done via a naturopath, nutritionist, or functional medicine practitioner.

During the last few years of my fertility journey, my approach was that if roughly 50% of the population had the MTHFR gene, then I was likely to be one of them as I had a history of infertility and recurrent pregnancy loss. So, I acted as if I had the MTHFR gene mutation in terms of my diet, lifestyle and supplement regime. When I conceived, my supplements included a prenatal multivitamin with activated B vitamins including folate and not folic acid, an additional supplement of 800 mcg 5-MTHFR plus methylcobalamin (active B12) because my B12 was low. A healthy methylation cycle involves the teamwork of both folate and vitamin B12, so I made sure I took optimal levels of both.

I encourage you to take advantage of the testing options that are available now, however, if you can't go down the testing route, then I would encourage you to act like you have the MTHFR gene mutation as well, especially if you have a history of unexplained infertility, recurrent pregnancy loss, and low thyroid function. 'People experiencing fertility problems and recurrent miscarriages have a strong likelihood to have the genetic variant that makes folic acid supplementation essentially useless—and that use of active folate in the form of 5-MTHF is beneficial.' [5]

As well as eating leafy green vegetables, avoiding foods with folic acid and taking a prenatal with active folate, you can also support methylation by:

- Eating a clean whole foods diet, organic, where possible

- Reducing refined sugar and processed foods

- Supporting your gut microbiome and digestive health

- Eliminating food sensitivities and inflammatory foods

- Exercising regularly

- Reducing your stress levels where you can.

Where can I find more information about the MTHFR gene mutation?

I've only touched on the basics when it comes to fertility problems. There is so much more reading you can do if you want to find out more about the MTHFR gene. Dr. Ben Lynch is the leading expert on MTHFR and has lots of information available on his website (www.mthfr.net) including a video course you can sign up to. I also recommend his book *Dirty Genes*, which is a very helpful resource.

To summarize, if you have a history of infertility, recurrent pregnancy loss, thyroid issues, or suspect that you have the MTHFR gene mutation, I strongly recommend that you:

- Consider getting tested by a nutritionist, naturopath, or functional medicine doctor

- Get rid of ALL folic acid and change to methylfolate (5-MTHFR)

- Check all your supplements for folic acid

- Take a prenatal multivitamin with activated B vitamins and NO folic acid

- As well as your prenatal multivitamin, you may need to take an additional supplement of 5-MTHFR, so you are taking at least 800 mcg of folate per day. Depending on your age and whether you have a MTHFR mutation, you may need more than this. If you are unsure, work with a practitioner. It would be wise to build up gradually as some people are sensitive to large doses of folate opening up previously blocked detoxification pathways. Start with a small dose and see how you respond

- Act like you have the MTHFR gene mutation in terms of your diet and lifestyle

Vitamin B12

Studies show that a deficiency in vitamin B12 plays a role in infertility and recurrent miscarriage, particularly early pregnancy loss before five weeks. A recent 2023 study concluded that a reduced serum B12, along with serum folic acid, was significantly associated with recurrent pregnancy loss cases and that 'Folic acid and vitamin B12 supplementation before next pregnancy in recurrent pregnancy loss patients is likely to be beneficial in improving pregnancy outcomes' [6]

Despite this, general practitioners and fertility specialists rarely include B12 in prenatal screening. During my 10-year journey with secondary infertility and recurrent pregnancy loss, no one tested my B12 levels at all. Yet vitamin B12 plays an important role in folate metabolism, and we all know how important folate is.

It was only later in my journey that I realised the significance of vitamin B12 and got myself tested. This was just after I had miscarried my IVF baby, as I felt at the time that my mind was foggy, and I couldn't concentrate on anything. My test results confirmed my B12 was low, and it was no wonder as I had so much blood drawn for blood tests during the period I was doing IVF. Vitamin B12 proved to be one of the missing links for me. When I finally got pregnant three years later, I needed high daily doses of B12 as methyl cobalamin to support my pregnancy.

So why is vitamin B12 so important?

Vitamin B12 is an essential nutrient that works together with folate in the synthesis of DNA, RNA, and red blood cells. Adequate levels of vitamin B12 are needed for methylation, folate metabolism and reducing homocysteine levels.

Homocysteine is an amino acid that is broken down by vitamin B12, B6 and folate to create other amino acids such as methionine and cysteine. High levels of homocysteine in the blood indicate that methylation is not working efficiently and that the body is likely to be deficient in the methyl donors B12, B6, and folate. These methylation nutrients are all necessary to prevent high levels of homocysteine levels in the blood and to reduce the risk of miscarriage. Taking a supplement with folate, B6 and B12 can help to reduce homocysteine levels.

Vitamin B12 also helps to boost the endometrium lining to prepare for implantation, which reduces the chances of implantation failure. It also helps to regulate brain activity and is involved in the production of the myelin sheath around the nerves and the conduction of nerve impulses.

What causes low B12?

Meat, fish, dairy products, and eggs are the best sources of vitamin B12. However, even if you consume meat a few times a day, your body can still become deficient if your body can't absorb it. Our gut bacteria can also manufacture vitamin B12 in the large intestines.

The absorption process of vitamin B12 is complex and `uptake depends on gastric parietal cells excreting hydrochloric acid, intrinsic factor, and pepsin. Pancreatic enzymes and receptors in the distal ileum must be present along with the blood protein transcobalamin II to process B12. Lastly, the liver converts B12 to the active forms adenosylcobalamin and methylcobalamin for utilization.' [7]

In order to absorb B12 from food, we must produce intrinsic factor, a protein that binds to B12 from food and transports it to the small intestines where it is absorbed into the bloodstream. Intrinsic factor is a mucoprotein enzyme produced by the parietal cells of the stomach, which also make hydrochloric acid. Any problems with the stomach, stress, inflammation, allergies, and aging can reduce the production of hydrochloric acid and intrinsic factor. So, for vitamin B12 to be absorbed, a person must have a healthy, efficient digestive system.

Common causes of vitamin B12 malabsorption:

- Leaky gut and inflammatory bowel disease

- Gut dysbiosis

- Low stomach acid, known as hypochlorhydria

- The autoimmune condition pernicious anaemia - as the body attacks and destroys intrinsic factor, the protein that is essential for B12 absorption

- Acid suppressant medications

- Excessive alcohol

- Vegan or vegetarian diets as plant sources of B12 have poor absorption.

According to various studies, 50% of long-term vegetarians and 80% of vegans are extremely low in B12. According to functional medicine practitioner and author Chris Kresser, 'B12 is the only vitamin that contains a trace element (cobalt), which is why it is called cobalamin. Animals produce cobalamin in their gut. It is the only vitamin we cannot get from plants or sunlight. Plants do not need vitamin B12, so they do not store it. A common myth amongst vegetarians and vegans is that it is possible to get vitamin B12 from plant sources like seaweed, fermented soy, spirulina, and brewer's yeast. But plant foods said to contain B12 contain B12 analogs called cobamides that block the intake of and increase the need for true B12.' [8]

Because the body stores vitamin B12, it can sometimes take about five years for some of the more severe symptoms to manifest.

Typical symptoms of B12 deficiency:

- Weakness, fatigue, tiredness, and feeling run down

- Poor memory, brain fog, light-headedness, and dizziness

- Depression (B12 is involved in the synthesis of serotonin and dopamine)

- Heart palpitations, shortness of breath

- Pale skin

- A smooth tongue

- Lack of appetite

- Constipation, diarrhoea, gas and bloating

- Numbness and tingling in the hands, legs, and feet (because of nerve damage)

- Muscle weakness and coordination problems

- Mental health issues such as depression, anxiety, memory loss, changes in behaviour

- Fertility issues and recurrent early miscarriage

If you have any of the symptoms listed above, it would be worth getting your B12 levels tested by your health practitioner, as you may need supplementation or B12 injections. If you are looking to take a B12 supplement, look for one that contains sublingual methylcobalamin, which is the active form of vitamin B12 that is more bioavailable than the common form cyanocobalamin. There are several brands available.

After you have been tested, make sure to ask your doctor for a copy of your results. To optimise fertility, pregnancy, and to reduce the risk of miscarriage, levels should be at least 500 pg/mL. Unfortunately, the normal range in New Zealand is lower than in other countries, with levels of 200 pg/mL and above being considered normal. Levels around 200 pg/mL are not optimal for pregnancy and preventing early pregnancy loss. An optimal range is 500 pg/mL or above.

Vitamin E

Vitamin E is a fat-soluble vitamin that is beneficial for both male and female fertility. Consider your vitamin E status if you have problems digesting and absorbing dietary fats; you have had your gallbladder removed, have coeliac disease and inflammatory bowel conditions such as Crohn's disease. Low levels of vitamin E are very common with coeliac disease. Vitamin E is a very important antioxidant that helps to protect cell membranes from free radical damage, so it has a protective role for both the sperm and the egg.

Important functions of vitamin E for fertility:

- It increases blood flow to the uterus, which helps to thicken the uterine lining

- Improves sperm health and motility

- Helps to regulate the menstrual cycle and reduce PMS symptoms

- Helps to prevent miscarriage

- Supports a healthy amniotic sac in pregnancy, which helps to protect against premature rupture and miscarriage

- Can increase success rates for IVF if taken as a supplement by both men and women

- Can boost circulation and decrease the tendency for blood clots

Vitamin E deficiency signs:

- Impaired immunity

- Vision problems

- Muscle weakness

- Balance problems

- Brain fog

- Digestive issues

- Skin rashes

- Hair loss

Good food sources of vitamin E are wheat germ, wheat germ oil, nuts, nut butter, seeds, rice bran oil, olive oil, avocado oil, barley, green leafy vegetables, broccoli, asparagus, avocados, kiwifruit, mangos, berries and tomatoes.

To absorb vitamin E, your liver, gallbladder and pancreas must be working efficiently to produce bile and pancreatic enzymes that emulsify and digest fats. Taking a digestive enzyme formula that contains ox bile with meals can be helpful if you have problems digesting fats or you have had your gallbladder removed.

If you decide to supplement with vitamin E, choose one with a mixture of tocopherols, as studies have shown they have a stronger effect compared to just alpha tocopherol in isolation.

Next steps

Here are three actions you can take to implement what you have learnt from this chapter:

1. Eat a balanced diet for fertility that is rich in coloured fruits and vegetables for antioxidants, healthy fats, proteins, fermented foods, nuts and seeds and gluten-free grains. Avoid processed foods, refined sugar, too much caffeine and alcohol.

2. As a foundational support, take a prenatal multivitamin for both men and women with activated B vitamins and choline.

3. Ensure you are taking at least 800 mcg of methylfolate and no folic acid from all other supplements. Consider testing for the MTHFR gene mutation, as you may need to take a higher dose. I recommend working with a qualified practitioner who can help organise testing and can recommend an appropriate supplement for your needs.

Chapter Four

Gut health and fertility

How we digest and absorb food has an influence on the health of every organ in the body, including the reproductive system. Approximately 70% of your immune system is located in your gut and your immune system plays an important role in your ability to get pregnant and to maintain a pregnancy. For many people, improving gut health is often the missing link with unexplained infertility.

How does digestion impact fertility?

A properly functioning digestive system breaks down food, absorbs nutrients, and eliminates toxins from the body that can affect fertility. A healthy digestive system ensures you are absorbing crucial nutrients for reproductive health. Even if you have a very healthy diet, if you are not digesting and absorbing the nutrients from your food efficiently, you will most likely have nutritional deficiencies which can lead to hormone imbalances and organ dysfunction.

Poor digestion can also lead to sluggish liver health, which can decrease the ability of the body to eliminate excess and harmful estrogens and toxins that can contribute to hormone imbalances. It may also contribute to low thyroid function, as beneficial gut bacteria are involved in the conversion of T4 (thyroxine) to T3 (triiodothyronine), which occurs in the liver.

Here are some of the most common signs of poor digestive function, although we can link many non-digestive symptoms to poor gut health as well:

- Bloating and gas

- Reflux and heartburn

- Abdominal pain

- Nausea

- Diarrhoea

- Constipation

- Greasy stools, which is a sign of poor fat absorption

- Skin problems

- Fatigue

- Yeast infections

- Gallbladder problems.

The importance of gut bacteria

The digestive system is home to over 500 different species of beneficial microbes and a healthy balance of your inner ecosystem is important for proper gut function. There are many things that can cause an imbalance in gut bacteria such as stress, a poor diet, high sugar intake, a lack of fibre, antibiotics and other medications.

Immune related fertility issues

In many cases, we can connect poor digestion to immune related fertility issues. This is because intestinal permeability, commonly referred to as leaky gut, can be the underlying cause of many autoimmune conditions and allergic reactions.

Intestinal permeability allows toxins and undigested foods to pass through the leaky gut wall into the bloodstream. This creates inflammation and sends alert messages to the immune system that there is an attack going on. If this happens every time you eat a food you are intolerant to, your immune system can become overreactive, triggered by substances that wouldn't normally be harmful.

A confused, overactive immune system may attack itself, causing inflammation and damage to body tissues. This is how many autoimmune conditions occur. It is challenging for a baby to thrive in this environment.

Here are some actions you can take to support your gut

Food intolerances

There are many options in New Zealand and worldwide for food intolerance testing ranging from a hair test, muscle testing, and an IgG blood spot test. It may be beneficial for you to consider consulting a naturopath, nutritionist, or functional medicine practitioner to guide you through the process of identifying and eliminating any food intolerances using a relevant testing approach. Avoiding reactive foods for a while will help to take some pressure off the immune system. If you choose not to pay for any testing, In the very least, consider cutting out or reducing inflammatory foods such as gluten, which has been linked in studies to fertility problems, dairy if you react to it, sugar, processed foods and alcohol.

Probiotic supplements

Take a beneficial probiotic supplement each day to enhance your gut microbiome. My favourite probiotics are the spore forming probiotics as I have had excellent results in clinic with clients with autoimmune conditions and allergies. Spore forming probiotic helps to heal intestinal permeability and support the immune system. Some of the beneficial spore forming strains are Bacillus Indicus HU36, Bacillus Subtilis HU58, Bacillus Coagulans SC-208, Bacillus Licheniformis SL-307 and Bacillus Clausii SC-109. These strains are all found in the Megasporebiotic from Microbiome Labs, which is the probiotic I take.

Fermented foods

Cultures around the world have been eating fermented foods for hundreds of years, especially in the days before refrigeration, as it was the only way to preserve vegetables. The process of fermentation creates a powerhouse of naturally occurring beneficial bacteria, much more than you would ever get from a probiotic supplement and much more affordable too.

Fermented foods are food items that have undergone a process of lacto fermentation, where natural bacteria consume the naturally present sugars and starches in the food, resulting in the production of lactic acid. This process preserves the food, making the food easier to digest, and creates colonies of beneficial bacteria which is so good for our digestive and immune health. I have heard reports of people with chronic allergies and health issues healing themselves by adopting a diet rich in fermented foods!

Great examples of fermented foods are home-made probiotic yoghurt, kefir, sauerkraut, and kombucha. I consider sauerkraut to be the king of fermented foods as it is so easy to make yourself at home. It is best to start off with a small teaspoon each day and build up gradually, as too much at once may cause uncomfortable digestive symptoms if you are not used to it.

How to make your own sauerkraut

You will need:

- A 2.5 litre mason jar with flip top lid that secures shut

- 1 whole cabbage (green or red although green is my favourite)

- Sea salt

- Caraway seeds (optional)

Directions:

1. Cut the cabbage in half, put the other half aside and slice the remaining half into very fine slithers.

2. Put the sliced half of the cabbage in a large bowl and add about 1 tablespoon of sea salt and 1 teaspoon caraway seeds.

3. Massage the sliced cabbage, seeds and salt like you are hand washing clothes, making sure the cabbage gets covered with the salt (you may need to add a little more). Keep massaging and squeezing the cabbage for about 5–10 minutes until it sweats a liquid.

4. Once you cannot get any more liquid out of it, separate the liquid from the cabbage and keep the liquid aside in another bowl. Place the cabbage at the bottom of the mason jar and tap down firmly so it is all squashed in at the bottom.

5. Repeat steps 1–4 with the remaining half of the cabbage. Firmly place the second half of the cabbage on top of the first half of the cabbage in the mason jar. Then pour all the cabbage juice over the top so the cabbage is sitting under the juice.

6. For the cabbage to ferment, it always needs to be under the surface of the juice. I like to put a weight on top of it, so it pushes it down into the juice. I used a small snap locked bag filled with water, but you could use a small dish or something else that helps to push the cabbage down.

7. Close the lid and leave it to ferment at room temperature on your kitchen bench or in your kitchen cupboard. In the first few days of the fermentation process, there will be a lot of bubbling going on and gasses forming in the jar. It is important that you open and close the lid quickly at least once or twice a day to release some gasses. If you forget to do this, your sauerkraut might explode.

8. Your sauerkraut will be ready in about five to seven days. When it is ready, transfer it to the fridge and enjoy. It will last up to six months in the fridge.

Gut healing meat stock

Meat stock is rich in gelatin and collagen, making it highly beneficial for gut health. Many consider it to be the "glue that heals and seals the intestinal lining." It is the principal healing food on the GAPS diet to support detoxification and to help heal and seal the gut wall.

Once or twice a week, make a gut healing meat stock. You can regularly consume the stock either on its own as a drink, or use as a base for soups, stews and casseroles.

I adapted the following meat stock recipe from Dr Natasha Campbell McBride's original recipe in her book *Gut and Psychology Syndrome*:

Meat stock is extremely nourishing and is full of vitamins, minerals, and amino acids and gelatin in bio available forms that are easy to absorb. Meat stock has been used for centuries as a healing folk remedy for the digestive system, as it supports digestion and heals the gut lining. The nourishment comes from the bone marrow, cartilage and other connective tissue. Aim to have one to two cups a day if you can.

How to make meat stock:

- To make meat stock, all you need is some meat with bones to make a good meat stock plus a large pot of water and salt and pepper. You can use beef, lamb, pork or chicken.

- For lamb, pork or beef, put the joints, bones and meat in a large pot. Add pepper and salt to taste and fill up the pot with water.

- Heat until it boils, then cover the pan and reduce the heat to the minimum and simmer for at least three hours. The longer you simmer the meat on the bones, the more they will give out to the stock and the more nourishing it will be.

- For chicken, put a whole or half of a chicken in a large pot. Fill it up with water, add salt and pepper and heat until it boils.

- Reduce the heat and simmer for two hours. Take the chicken out of the pot and put the stock through a sieve. Alternatively, you can leave the meat in a slow cooker to cook for the day.

Prebiotic foods

Eat prebiotic foods to feed your beneficial bacteria. Prebiotic foods are non-digestible fibre foods that pass through the stomach and small intestines without being broken down by stomach acid and digestive enzymes. As prebiotic foods can't be broken down, they reach the colon where they feed our beneficial gut bacteria. Some prebiotic foods to include in your diet are chicory root, unripe banana, onions, garlic, asparagus, dandelion greens, and Jerusalem artichoke.

Apple cider vinegar

Have a glass of warm water with a tablespoon of apple cider vinegar 20 minutes before meals and first thing in the morning. This encourages the production of stomach acid, which helps the body to digest and absorb protein better. Apple cider vinegar also helps to cleanse the liver. As an alternative, half a freshly squeezed lemon in warm water also encourages the production of stomach acid.

Digestive enzymes

Many people have poor digestive function, although they may not realise it. Our saliva, stomach, and pancreas naturally produce digestive enzymes to help us break down and absorb carbohydrates, fats, proteins, and lactose. Our production of digestive enzymes naturally decreases as we age and can be even more deficient if you have chronic in-flammatory or allergic conditions. Supplementing with digestive enzymes with meals can provide your body with the tools to break down and absorb your foods properly, which can help to reduce symptoms such as gas, bloating, constipation and diarrhoea.

For gluten and casein digestion, some digestive enzymes are more effective than others. If you eat gluten and casein (from milk) but find you have trouble digesting it, then you may wish to take a digestive enzyme formula that contains the enzyme DPP- IV, although not all of them have it. This will help you digest and assimilate the problematic proteins found in gluten and casein, which for many are difficult to digest, and regular consumption can lead to intestinal inflammation.

DPP-IV is a proteolytic enzyme that can break down the problematic proteins that contribute to gluten and casein intolerance. It allows the proteins to be absorbed safely in their digested state. If you have coeliac disease, the autoimmune condition where gluten consumption damages the lining of the gut, you will need to avoid gluten permanently. If you accidentally consume gluten, the DPP-IV enzymes in your SOS kit can help to reduce symptoms, but you should not rely on them to consume gluten.

L-glutamine

The amino acid l-glutamine promotes the regeneration and repair of the enterocyte cells of the intestinal lining. It helps to re-establish the integrity of the mucosal lining, which prevents toxins and undigested foods from passing into the bloodstream. Taking 1 -5 grams daily on an empty stomach is beneficial for healing and repairing the intestinal lining.

Mindful eating

It is important to practice mindful eating to give your digestive system the optimal environment to digest food. Where possible, sit at the dinner table in a relaxed state and chew your food at least 15–20 times. Take the time to enjoy the taste and the smell of the food, which helps to stimulate digestive juices. Avoid eating on the run, as this will lead to food not being chewed properly, which will put extra strain on your digestive system.

Bitter foods

Bitter foods and herbs are crucial to your health as the bitter taste helps to stimulate stomach acid, digestive enzymes, and bile flow, which supports the digestion and absorption of nutrients from food.

Unfortunately, most people are not getting enough bitter foods as it is common for people to neglect bitter tastes in favour of more appealing choices like sweet or salty. This causes a problem, as not only are bitter foods important for digestion, but they also support liver detoxification through their sulfur-containing compounds. According to

Ayurvedic tradition, bitter foods reduce cravings and aid in weight loss, so it is important to have at least one serving a day of bitter foods with meals.

Examples of bitter foods are kale, dandelion, watercress, parsley, radish, leafy greens, bitter melon, and basil. A simple way to ensure you are getting a daily supply of bitter foods in your diet is to have a handful of mesclun leaves with each meal. You can grab a bag of mesclun all year round from most supermarkets and fruit and vegetable retailers.

The GAPS Diet

After training to be a certified GAPS practitioner in 2015, I also spent periods of time on and off the GAPS Diet when I felt I needed some extra support. After having IVF, which sadly ended in a miscarriage at six weeks, I completed the GAPS Introduction Diet for about six weeks as a reset. I felt my hormones were out of balance after the IVF and I felt depleted in nutrients after having so many blood tests. I also spent time on and off the Full GAPS Diet when I felt my health was not optimal and my gut needed some healing. Prior to conceiving, I had been on the GAPS Introduction Diet for about four weeks before transitioning to the Full GAPS Diet.

What is the GAPS Diet?

The GAPS Diet is a comprehensive gut healing protocol developed by Dr Natasha Campbell-McBride, a UK based neurologist and nutritionist who used the GAPS nutritional protocol to help heal her son from autism. She then coached her clients through the same diet to assist with the healing of many conditions, such as autism, ADD/ADHD, dyspraxia, dyslexia, depression, allergies, eczema, asthma, hormone issues and autoimmune diseases.

GAPS stands for *Gut and Psychology Syndrome* and *Gut and Physiology Syndrome*, which are the names of Dr Natasha's best-selling books. Both books establish a connection between the health of the gut and the health of the brain and the rest of the body. Dr Natasha recognised that the key to treating many disorders is to get to the root cause, which is always COMPROMISED GUT HEALTH.

The GAPS protocol focuses on healing foods, supplements, detoxification, reducing toxic load and cleaning up your environment. The temporary diet encourages consuming an abundance of traditional healing foods such as nourishing meat stock, meats, organ meat, soups, fermented foods, non-starchy vegetables, nuts, seeds, raw honey, raw vegetable juices and beneficial fats. It is also important to reduce foods that irritate the gut lining and cause inflammation such as grains, sugar and starchy vegetables.

There are two parts to the GAPS diet: the *Introduction Diet* and the *Full GAPS Diet*. The Introduction Diet is beneficial for individuals with severe symptoms, digestive disorders, allergies, and diarrhoea, as it accelerates the healing and sealing of the gut wall, resulting in a faster recovery.

There are six stages to the Introduction Diet, and you can move through the stages at your own pace, determined by your symptoms. As the gut heals, you introduce new foods stage by stage until you reach a point that you can begin the Full GAPS Diet. People who find the introduction diet too restrictive, or have chronic constipation, may be better off starting with the Full GAPS Diet as it is higher in fibre. Depending on your symptoms, you may benefit from being on the Full GAPS Diet for up to two years. All grains and starchy vegetables are eliminated on the Full GAPS Diet because they can irritate the gut.

The GAPS Diet is temporary gut healing protocol rather than a permanent way of living, although many people integrate the GAPS principles into their way of life. I certainly did that as the GAPS Diet principles aligned with the principles of the Weston A. Price Foundation. My diet included plenty of beneficial fats, fermented foods, cultured dairy, meat broth, organic meat, organ meat, vegetables, fruits, nuts, and seeds.

The GAPS protocol is a gut healing journey that can be challenging at times, so if you can it is best to get the support and guidance from your local certified GAPS practitioner.

The official GAPS website lists all the practitioners by region so you can find one local to you. There are certified GAPS practitioners located all over the world as well as certified GAPS coaches who can help provide guidance with the food preparation. A certified GAPS practitioner has been trained by Dr Natasha Campbell-McBride, so has the experience and knowledge to help develop a GAPS protocol that is suited to your individual needs and to provide ongoing support and advice. The international GAPS practitioner listing is found on the official GAPS website: www.gaps.me.

Gluten and fertility

There have been several studies linking gluten to infertility and recurrent miscarriage. This is because gluten is inflammatory for many people and can cause damage to the lining of the small intestine. Over time this can lead to the development of coeliac disease in some people (which can often go undiagnosed) as well as other autoimmune issues that could contribute to infertility.

Experts estimate that up to 80% of people with coeliac disease do not experience obvious digestive symptoms, resulting in the condition often remaining undetected. This was certainly the case with me, which is why I advise my clients with unexplained infertility and recurrent miscarriages to try a gluten-free diet for at least six months to see if it helps. Fertility specialists do not routinely test for coeliac disease until you have had several miscarriages, then they will test you for various autoimmune conditions. This is often when doctors uncover coeliac disease.

I am not suggesting that everyone who is trying to get pregnant needs to avoid gluten, as this is not the case. However, if you have been trying to conceive for a while, if you have been labelled as unexplained, or if you are about to undergo IVF, then trying a gluten-free diet to increase your chances would be a good idea. When your body is inflamed from gluten or other food intolerances, then the body is also in a state of stress, which alerts your body that there is an emergency going on and it is not a good time to get pregnant.

Here are some of the key findings from research on coeliac disease and infertility:

A study found that non-coeliac gluten sensitivity can induce malabsorption of key nutrients required for fertility such as iron, folate, zinc and vitamin B12. This is because inflammation of the lining of the small intestines caused by gluten can damage our enterocyte cells that absorb nutrients from our food, which leads to nutritional deficiencies. [1]

Another study could detect a significantly increased prevalence (5.9%) of undiagnosed coeliac disease among women presenting with unexplained infertility. The findings suggest the importance of screening infertile female patients, particularly those with unexplained infertility, for coeliac disease. [2]

A 2014 study came to a similar conclusion. Physicians should investigate women with unexplained infertility, recurrent miscarriage, and intrauterine growth restriction for undiagnosed coeliac disease. Women with coeliac disease show an increased risk of miscarriage, intrauterine growth restriction, low birth weight and preterm delivery. However, the risk is significantly reduced by a gluten-free diet. [3]

Another 2016 study found that up to 50% of women with untreated coeliac disease refer to an experience of miscarriage or an unfavourable outcome of pregnancy. Despite this, coeliac disease is still little considered during the evaluation of infertility. [4]

A report studied the effect of coeliac disease and its treatment on fertility and pregnancy in 74 patients. Those on a normal diet had a shorter reproductive period, were relatively infertile, and had a higher incidence of spontaneous abortions than those on a gluten-free diet. Although maternal health did not appear to be seriously impaired by pregnancy in undiagnosed coeliacs, those on a gluten-free diet had significantly fewer symptoms and had heavier babies. [5]

A 2018 study found that prior to the diagnosis of coeliac disease, an increased risk of adverse pregnancy outcomes was seen, whereas after the diagnosis and the adoption of a gluten-free diet, no influence on reproductive outcomes was found. The study found that prior to being diagnosed, coeliac disease women have an extra risk of spontaneous abortion equal to 11 extra spontaneous abortions per 1000 pregnancies and 1.62 extra stillbirths per 1000 pregnancies compared to the non-coeliac disease women. [6]

Some cases of infertility, IVF failure and recurrent miscarriage may be because of an overreactive immune system reacting to a high percentage of natural killer cells, which are linked to recurrent miscarriage and implantation failure. A study of natural killer cells in the lab and in mice found that exposure to gliadin (the protein in gluten) increased natural killer cell presence, toxicity, and activity. No researchers have conducted current studies on humans. [7]

Is it necessary for you to adopt a gluten-free diet?

If your fertility issues are unexplained and you have been trying to conceive for a while without success, then removing gluten from your diet may be worth considering. Especially if you have other underlying health issues going on, such as hormone imbalances, autoimmune disease, allergies, or digestive issues. If you are planning to go through a cycle of IVF, then it would be beneficial to go on a gluten free diet at least three months prior to the IVF treatment to reduce any risk of inflammation.

My gut health story

I probably have had coeliac disease for most of my life, but it was only in my early thirties that I found out for sure and since then I have been completely gluten free.

There is a history of autoimmune disease in my family, with my dad, auntie and late grandmother suffering from various autoimmune conditions. My late grandfather experienced frequent stomach pain, but it wasn't a topic my family was comfortable discussing openly.

My mother didn't breastfeed me as a baby because it wasn't a popular practice in the UK during the 1970s. During my first three months of life, I suffered from colic and would scream for hours. As a child, I developed asthma before the age of 10; I was very underweight and would often have stomach bugs and bouts of nausea and diarrhoea. According to my dad, I was a very fussy eater and would only want to eat white bread!

In my twenties, I continued with my unhealthy lifestyle by binge drinking alcohol every weekend. I was a season ticket holder of our local football club Southampton, so we would drink beer from 12pm to 2am the next morning and would do that most weekends!

During my mid-twenties, I developed a skin rash after using a gym jacuzzi that refused to heal. My doctor prescribed me several courses of antibiotics to heal the rash, which caused my health to deteriorate further as I ended up being on antibiotics for almost two months. I didn't take probiotics during this time, as there was still a lack of awareness during the early 2000s.

It was during this period that I started experiencing dermatitis hepiformis, a rash that is associated with gluten intake. Unfortunately, dermatologists in the UK were unaware of this connection and continued to treat me with steroids and antibiotics.

When I was 25, I paid to have a food intolerance test through York Laboratories in the UK. The test identified gluten as a severe intolerance and recommended removing it from my diet, as well as a few other foods. I was young and tried my best to minimize gluten (probably around 80%), but I couldn't resist the occasional indulgence in baking and pizza, continuing this habit for the next seven years. I guess I didn't really know what I know now or care so much because I was still quite young, so my rash continued. Despite this, I didn't have any apparent symptoms affecting my stomach.

At age 32, I gave birth to my son (who at the time of writing this is 15) and then my health deteriorated. Although I was eating a healthy diet and studying nutrition, I was still not 100% gluten free, and it was only when I struggled to conceive a second child that I realised the impact gluten had been having on my health. I still looked seven months pregnant for about two years after his birth and had anemia (low iron and B12), fatigue and very dark circles under my eyes. My rash continued, and the only way I could keep this under control was with steroid cream.

In 2011, my doctor tested me for various autoimmune diseases to investigate my fertility problems and I finally found out that I had coeliac disease. From that point onwards, I never again touched gluten. Within two weeks my bloating disappeared, my rash took about six months to clear, and I gradually started to feel a bit more human again as my damaged gut repaired and I could start absorbing nutrients again.

In 2014, my son, who was age six at the time, was told by his teacher that he may have dyslexia. Researching this condition led to me to discover the *Gut and Psychology Syndrome (GAPS)* protocol. In 2015, I had the privilege of attending a two-day intensive training on the GAPS protocol in Sydney with Dr. Natasha Campbell McBride. The amazing knowledge I gained from this intensive two-day training transformed my health, my family's health, and my clinic.

I spent the next two years on the Full GAPS Diet, and it was a real game changer with my healing journey. Most of my symptoms, including asthma, improved significantly. My son's issue with dyslexia also quickly resolved after being on a semi-Full GAPS Diet, and his schoolteachers never spoke about it again.

As a nutritionist, I frequently support clients as they work through the GAPS protocol to heal their gut lining. In order to fully grasp the correct approach and the challenges clients face, I completed the GAPS Introduction Diet twice. Interestingly, I was on the GAPS Introduction Diet for four weeks (before transitioning to the Full GAPS Diet) when I discovered I was pregnant naturally at age 43 after 10 long years of secondary infertility. I was making a lot of other changes at the time, like quitting a stressful job and changing supplements, so I don't know for sure if the Introduction Diet was the reason I got pregnant, but I like to think it played a huge part. During my time on the Introduction Diet, I felt I had so much more energy. I really felt nourished and healthy.

Testing for coeliac disease

If you suspect you may have issues with gluten and you are still eating it daily, I recommend asking your doctor to test you for coeliac disease, the autoimmune condition that causes damage and inflammation to the small intestines following consumption of gluten. Autoimmune conditions put extra stress on the immune system and may well be affecting your ability to conceive and maintain a pregnancy. It is a good idea to rule out coeliac disease while you are still consuming gluten regularly, as this will enable the detection of coeliac antibodies in your blood test. It is harder to get a positive test if you are already avoiding gluten, which gives a false sense of security that gluten is fine for you. In all the times I was seeing specialists in both England and New Zealand for my skin rash, they did not test me for coeliac disease.

An important point to remember is that many people are not actually coeliac, but gluten can still cause inflammation and damage to the body. This is called non coeliac gluten sensitivity. If your doctor has ruled out coeliac disease, but you still feel you are having problems with gluten, food intolerance testing through a practitioner like myself can be a good way to identify intolerances.

The elimination test

If you are not keen on formal testing, try going completely gluten free for four weeks and then reintroduce wheat bread daily for four days to gauge how your body reacts. If you have any noticeable symptoms, this is a sign that you need to eliminate gluten for at least six months, possibly longer. The only issue with doing this is that if you decide at a later date to have screening for coeliac disease, it may show up negative as you have been avoiding all gluten. So, I would recommend having tests for coeliac disease with your doctor first, and if it is negative but you still feel gluten is a problem, then do the elimination test. Coeliac disease affects a small percentage of the population, but a larger percentage experience symptoms of non-coeliac gluten sensitivity.

Whether you have coeliac disease or non-coeliac gluten sensitivity, gluten is still damaging your body so avoiding gluten 100% is the key, something I learnt the hard way.

Next steps

Here are three actions you can take to implement the key points from this chapter:

1. If you experience digestive symptoms like bloating, gas, abdominal pain, diarrhea, and constipation, your gut requires some attention. Poor digestion may mean that you are not digestion and absorbing your food properly, which could lead to nutritional deficiencies that may affect fertility. The recommendations in this chapter, such as digestive enzymes, probiotics, regular meat stock to heal the gut lining and fermented foods, are a good place to start.

2. If you have an autoimmune condition, or suffer from infertility or recurrent pregnancy loss, then consider going gluten free, as many studies have linked gluten consumption to infertility and recurrent miscarriage.

3. Work with a practitioner to investigate and eliminate food intolerances. If you are reacting to any foods, even healthy foods, then this could trigger the immune system to overreact, which could lead to unwanted inflammation in the body. A body that is inflamed is not in the best condition to conceive.

Chapter Five

Finding hormone harmony

A healthy balance of hormones is extremely important for reproductive health. I love this quote from Dr Susanne Esche-Belke and Dr Suzann Kirschner-Browns in their book *Our Hormones Our Health* as it really describes how important hormones are to our health as they are involved in many functions of the body.

"Hormones dictate our daily rhythm, stabilise our immune system, keep our brain fit, strengthen our bones, stimulate our digestion and blood circulation, and regulate our appetite and core body temperature. They steer muscle and bone growth, the menstrual cycle, our feelings, our moods, and countless other elements of our physical and mental experience."

The key to good hormones is a healthy balance, as too much or too little of a certain hormone can affect our health, especially fertility. Most hormones work as a team, so if one is not performing well, the entire team is affected. It can be difficult to get an accurate understanding of your hormone levels, as the standard blood tests offered by doctors and fertility clinics may not reveal the whole story.

In this chapter, I am going to focus on the common hormone imbalances that affect fertility, how to get further testing done if you resonate with any of these hormone profiles, and what you can do naturally to help restore hormone harmony.

Estrogen dominance

Estrogen dominance is a hormone imbalance that affects as many as 70% of women over the age of 35 and beyond. It occurs when there is either an excess of estrogen circulating through the body or when there is a dominance of estrogen compared to progesterone. Estrogen can also become problematic if there is too much of one type of estrogen compared to the other types of estrogen. Estrogen dominance can be a factor in infertility and recurrent pregnancy loss and so should always be evaluated as part of a preconception screening programme. I will discuss testing later in this chapter.

Estrogen is a key player in the regulation of the reproductive system. Estrogen is made in the ovaries, fat cells, adrenal glands, and the liver. There are three types of estrogen, and these will fluctuate depending on the stage of life you are at:

- *Estrone (E1)* - is dominant after menopause when your body stops making estradiol (E2) and estriol (E3)

- *Estradiol (E2)* – is the dominant type of estrogen in women from when they start menstruating through to menopause

- *Estriol (E3)* – is increased during pregnancy.

Estrogen will typically fluctuate during the menstrual cycle. It is low during menstruation and gradually rises during the follicular phase (days 1 – 14 if you have a 28-day cycle) reaching a peak at ovulation. The role of estrogen is to prepare the lining of the uterus for conception if it occurs. After its peak at ovulation, estrogen levels gradually decline during the luteal phase (the phase between ovulation and your period) as progesterone takes over as the dominant hormone. There are two typical patterns with estrogen dominance:

1. The body makes too much estrogen

2. Estrogen is high in relation to progesterone. This means there is not enough progesterone to balance out estrogen levels during the luteal phase

Symptoms of estrogen dominance:

- Premenstrual syndrome (PMS)

- Mood changes

- Breast tenderness and swelling

- Heavy periods

- Period pain

- Irregular periods

- Water retention

- Hair loss

- Weight gain and increased belly fat

- Bloating

- Reduced libido

Estrogen dominance can be the root cause of conditions such as infertility, miscarriage, endometriosis, fibroids, and thyroid dysfunction, as high levels of estrogen may affect thyroid hormone production.

Let's start by focusing on what we can do if you have the first pattern of estrogen dominance, which is when your body makes too much estrogen.

The importance of the liver

Estrogen metabolism is connected to the healthy functioning of the liver and whether the body is recycling excess and harmful estrogens or detoxifying them from the body. The liver converts estrogen into a water-soluble form so that it can be detoxified from the body. If your liver is not functioning optimally, rather than being eliminated, estrogen is recycled back into the bloodstream, leading to estrogen dominance. This is often what is happening when someone has excess estrogen circulating in the body.

Here are a few suggestions of how to support your liver so that it can clear estrogen effectively:

- Eat foods rich in sulforaphane, a compound found in broccoli or broccoli sprouts. Sulforaphane enhances sulfation, which is a liver detoxification pathway that helps with the clearance of estrogen. I often recommend broccoli sprouts in supplement form.

- Consume lightly cooked brassica vegetables daily, such as broccoli, kale, cauliflower, and cabbage, as they contain a substance called di-indolylmethane (DIM), which helps to promote healthy estrogen metabolism. DIM supports the liver to maintain normal estrogen levels, so it is useful if you have high levels of less desirable estrogen. You can also take DIM as a supplement, which is what I took to help with my estrogen dominance when I was trying to conceive. I took DIM until I found out I was pregnant and then stopped.

Gut health

The liver converts estrogen into a form that the gut can eliminate through the process of conjugation. It is then up to a healthy gut to eliminate the estrogen from the body and regular bowel motions are extremely important for this to happen. Constipation and poor gut health undo the conjugation process, recycling the estrogen back into the bloodstream, which increases estrogen levels.

It is also important that our gut flora is optimal, as an imbalance of gut flora can increase estrogen levels. Have you heard of the estrobolome? This is a relatively new term which establishes a connection between our gut microbiome and the regulation of estrogen. According to Aviva Romm, the estrobolome is 'a unique microbiome within your gut microbiome, made up of a collection of bacteria with special genes that help you metabolise estrogen.'[1]

It is amazing to think that our gut microbes play a role in regulating estrogen levels. An imbalance of gut bacteria can increase the production of an enzyme called beta-glucuronidase, which has a negative effect on estrogen metabolism by reducing the ability of the liver to detoxify estrogen, allowing the estrogen to be recycled into the bloodstream.

According to author and functional medicine practitioner Chris Kresser 'Microbes in the estrobolome produce beta-glucuronidase, an enzyme that deconjugates estrogen back into their active forms. Beta-glucuronidase activity produces active unbound estrogen that is capable of binding to estrogen receptors and influencing estrogen dependent physiological processes.' [2]

We can help protect against this by supplementing with calcium D-glucarate, which is a combination of glucaric acid and calcium, that helps to inhibit beta-glucuronidase. You can purchase calcium D-glucarate on its own as a powder or it can often be found in a supplement with DIM.

So, you can see the importance of maintaining a delicate balance of gut microbiome and estrobolome. There are many things that can affect this balance, including genetics, age, weight, diet, alcohol use, and environmental toxins. We can support our estrobolome by:

- Drinking plenty of water – aim for 30mls for each KG of body weight daily.

- Eat plenty of fibre from fruits and vegetables (5 – 8 servings a day).

- Eat prebiotic foods such as garlic, onions, leeks, unripe bananas, and asparagus to provide fuel for our beneficial bacteria. Prebiotic foods are non-digestible fibre foods that pass through the stomach and small intestines without being broken down by stomach acid and enzymes. As we cannot break prebiotic foods down, they reach the colon, where they feed our beneficial gut bacteria. They are fuel for our beneficial bacteria to thrive.

- Eat probiotic foods such as kefir, sauerkraut, kimchi and kombucha. Probiotic foods provide billions of naturally occurring beneficial gut microbes.

- Eating a range of polyphenol rich foods such as berries, grapes, spinach, broccoli, orange, dark chocolate, and green tea helps to feed our beneficial gut microbes and increase our microbiome diversity. Polyphenols contain antioxidants that have prebiotic and anti-microbial properties.

- Eliminate refined sugar, processed foods, and excess alcohol.

- Eat for the seasons.

- Rotate your foods for increased variety, which helps with microbiome diversity. Try not to have the same foods every day.

Xenoestrogens

We also have to be aware of xenoestrogens, which are endocrine disruptors that alter the normal function of hormones and mimic estrogen. We are exposed to xenoestrogens from everyday items around the house, such as plastic drink bottles and containers, pesticides, household cleaning chemicals, unfiltered drinking water, and personal care products such as cosmetics, skin creams, sunscreen, and sanitary items.

'Xenoestrogens are foreign estrogens, substances that are close enough in molecular structure to estrogen that they can bind to estrogen receptor sites with potentially hazardous outcomes.' [3]

It is difficult to remove all xenoestrogens completely since they come from multiple environmental sources. However, there are a few things we can do to reduce our exposure. These are:

- Choose organic, locally grown fruit and vegetables that are in season

- Buy organic meat, poultry, and dairy products to avoid added hormones and pesticides

- Avoid all pesticides, herbicides, and fungicides

- Reduce the use of plastics around the home, use glass rather than plastic containers

- Do not microwave food in plastic containers

- Avoid the use of plastic wrap to cover food where possible

- Avoid drinking from a plastic water bottle and never leave it in the sun or in a hot car

- Use natural chemical free laundry and household cleaning products

- Select natural tampons, pads, and toilet paper that are unbleached and chlorine free

- Filter drinking water

- Choose natural creams, cosmetics, soaps, and toothpaste that do not contain estrogenic chemicals

- Avoid nail polish and nail polish remover unless you find a natural brand.

The impact of stress on hormone balance

Let's now focus on the second estrogen dominance pattern, which is when estrogen is high in relation to progesterone but is not in excess in the body. This is known as relative estrogen dominance.

High estrogen levels in relation to progesterone is often associated with stress and the activity of the hypothalamic-pituitary-adrenal (HPA) axis, which involves the interaction between the hypothalamus, pituitary gland, and adrenal glands. The HPA axis regulates the body's adaptive response to stress.

HPA axis dysfunction (or adrenal fatigue, which is otherwise known) is when our adrenal glands function below normal levels, usually because of prolonged chronic stress. The adrenal glands are situated on top of the kidneys and regulate our stress response by producing stress hormones such as cortisol (long-term) and adrenaline (short-term) in response to stress. Long-term stress can lead to the depletion of the adrenal glands and can cause imbalances in the production of cortisol. When the body is in a long-term stress state, non-essential functions that are not important for immediate survival, such as the digestive system, reproduction system, and thyroid, start to slow down and down regulate.

Stress is an enormous factor, as it can interfere with our reproductive hormones, especially progesterone and testosterone, which are important hormones for fertility and pregnancy.

Progesterone is not only produced by the corpus luteum of the ovary but also by the adrenal glands. This means that if you are under a lot of stress, then your adrenal glands may have shut down your production of progesterone in favour of stress hormones such as cortisol and adrenaline. This is a reason why you may have low progesterone, especially after an anovulatory cycle where you may not have ovulated, which leads to relative estrogen dominance. I really believe this was a huge factor in my fertility journey and is likely to be similar to many women in this day and age. When we are under stress, our body shuts down our reproductive hormones, as getting pregnant is not considered essential for our survival. 'The stress response serves to prioritise survival over less essential physiological functions, including growth, and reproduction.' [4]

The priority is to focus on stress management and increasing progesterone to balance estrogen levels, while also supporting the liver and gut to support the detoxification of estrogen. I will explore stress and adrenal function in more detail in chapter seven.

Low estrogen

As well as estrogen dominance, low levels of estrogen can also affect fertility by impairing ovulation. This is because without adequate estrogen, the lining of the uterus is not a healthy thickness for a fertilised egg to implant.

Low estrogen can be a factor with perimenopausal women as estrogen levels naturally decline with age so if you are trying to conceive over the age of 40 it is important to consider this and get a DUTCH test completed looking at your whole hormone picture. Later in this chapter, I will explain more about DUTCH testing.

Excessive exercise, strict dieting, and being underweight can cause low estrogen, as well as thyroid and pituitary issues. Here are the typical symptoms of low estrogen:

- Vaginal dryness and a lack of cervical mucus

- Breast tenderness

- Mood changes, anxiety

- Night sweats and hot flashes

- Irregular cycles

- Insomnia

- Dry skin

- Brain fog

- Abdominal weight gain.

Support for low estrogen

Foods rich in phytoestrogens such as flaxseeds, lentils, chickpeas, pumpkin seeds, sunflower seeds, organic soy and almonds, can have estrogen-like effects on the body and may reduce symptoms.

A concept called seed cycling may be helpful for balancing hormones. This involves eating raw ground flaxseeds and pumpkin seeds from day 1 – 14 of your cycle to support estrogen production. Raw ground sunflower and sesame seeds are recommended from days 15–28 of your cycle to enhance progesterone production.

Taking omega-3, B vitamins, and zinc supplements can be beneficial, along with stress reduction, good sleep, and moderate exercise.

Isoflavones in red clover tea, a plant from the legume family, have a mild estrogenic effect. Drinking red clover tea during the follicular phase of the cycle can support estrogen levels and enhance ovulation.

Supporting healthy progesterone levels

Progesterone is a very important hormone for getting pregnant, maintaining a pregnancy and for female hormone health in general.

After ovulation, the corpus luteum of the ovaries produces progesterone to maintain a potential pregnancy. If there is no pregnancy, progesterone levels naturally decline until you get your menstrual period. If you are fortunate enough to be pregnant, progesterone levels continue to rise to maintain this.

Progesterone levels decline naturally from about age 35, so if you are of this age group and older, it is important that you are supporting your body's own production of progesterone with hormone building foods, nutrients, stress management and natural supplements. Here are some of the common symptoms of low progesterone:

- Premenstrual syndrome (PMS)

- Irregular periods

- Shorter cycles of around 24 days

- Headaches

- Mood changes, depression, or anxiety

- Hot flashes

- Bloating, weight gain

- Swollen and tender breasts

- Sleep issues

- Infertility

Fortunately, there are many diet and lifestyle suggestions that we can adopt to help support healthy progesterone levels:

Reduce stress

Try to reduce stress and make space for a baby in your life. If you have too many projects on the go, cut back. It is important that your future baby knows you have the time and the energy for it.

Try yoga and meditation and have a relaxing bath with a few drops of lavender essential oil added to the bath water. Deal with any health issues that you have that are causing stress to your body and mind.

DUTCH hormone testing

If you are over 40, avoid wasting time trying different supplements. Go straight for the DUTCH hormone test through a practitioner, then you know what you are dealing with. Depending on your test results, you may benefit from some nutritional and herbal supplements that can support a healthy balance of hormones. It is best to work with a qualified practitioner to find the best hormonal support for you.

DIM (di-indolylmethane)

As discussed earlier, you can support your liver's detoxification of estrogen by including plenty of brassica vegetables such as broccoli, cauliflower, kale, Brussels sprouts, and cabbage in your diet. They contain a substance called di-indolylmethane (DIM), which helps your liver detoxify excess estrogens by converting estrogen into a water-soluble form that the liver can detoxify.

If you have thyroid issues, lightly steam brassica vegetables rather than eating them raw. This is because raw brassica vegetables contain active goitrogens, a naturally occurring compound that can block the thyroid gland's absorption of iodine.

Ground linseed

Add one tablespoon of freshly ground linseed to smoothies or breakfast cereal. Linseed (otherwise known as flaxseed) contains lignans, a phytochemical that can help to balance estrogen and progesterone. Lignans can also help to lengthen a short luteal phase, which is the time between ovulation and your period.

Research has shown that lignans from linseed increase levels of sex hormone binding globulin (SHBG), a glycoprotein that binds excess estrogen and makes it inactive. So, it helps balance out any estrogen dominance by helping the body eliminate harmful or excess estrogens.

Ground linseed is great to include in your diet regularly to help balance hormones. If you want to be more specific, you can also do seed cycling, which is eating freshly ground seeds at certain times in your cycle for the effect they have on hormone production.

According to seed cycling experts, eating raw ground sunflower and sesame seeds on days 15–28 of your cycle can increase progesterone levels. I haven't personally tried it because of my preference for flexibility, but based on research, seed cycling seems like it could be quite beneficial.

Reduce exposure to xenoestrogens

As discussed earlier in this chapter, try to reduce your exposure to xenoestrogens from the environment. Where possible avoid the use of plastics (drink bottles, lunch boxes) solvents and adhesives (paint, nail polish, household cleaners) non-organic meats (they contain hormones to help them grow quickly) pesticides, herbicides, fungicides, emulsifiers in soap and cosmetics, and PCBs (polychlorinated biphenyl) from industrial waste.

Multivitamin

Take a quality prenatal multivitamin with activated B vitamins to ensure you are getting the essential nutrients to support your hormones and liver function. The multivitamin should contain at least 800 mcg of active methylfolate to support methylation and not synthetic folic acid.

Avoid any foods that stress the body, such as refined sugar, caffeine, alcohol, processed foods, and gluten. Caffeine is a stress for the adrenals and elevates cortisol.

Vitamin B6

Eat foods rich in vitamin B6 as it helps to regulate the hormones estrogen and progesterone. Vitamin B6 is very supportive if you have a luteal phase defect as it helps to increase progesterone levels and adequate progesterone levels are necessary for preparing the endometrium for the fertilised ovum. Optimal vitamin B6 levels are also important for methylation and liver detoxification.

Foods that are rich in vitamin B6 are chicken, pork, eggs, banana, liver, salmon, sweet-corn, Brussel sprouts, spinach, capsicum, garlic, cauliflower, celery, cabbage, broccoli, brewer's yeast, and wholegrain cereals.

Eat enough fat

Ensure you are eating enough fat in your diet, as healthy fat is essential for manufacturing hormones. If you are eating a low-fat diet, you may not be ovulating as your body may struggle without the building blocks to make important reproductive hormones, such as progesterone. I see this a lot in my clinic, as many of my female clients don't eat enough dietary fats. I think as a society we are still afraid of eating fat, after being conditioned with the "fat is bad" message for so long from public health agencies over the previous few decades. The problem is fat is so critical for fertility and if you are not eating enough, you may not be ovulating. A lack of fat will also affect the function of all your cells, organs, and tissues, so it is not an ideal environment for conception. If you are trying to conceive, I recommend having a healthy fat source with every meal (breakfast, lunch and dinner). Some good choices are:

- Avocado

- Deep sea oily fish such as salmon, tuna, mackerel and sardines

- Full fat organic dairy products – organic milk, raw milk, butter, cheese, yoghurt and kefir

- Olive oil, flaxseed oil, hempseed oil

- Meat and poultry fat

- Meat stock

- Nuts and seeds

- Coconut cream, coconut oil

Sleep

For a healthy balance of hormones, it is important to prioritise sleep. Aim to be in bed by 10 pm at least three times a week, as sleep deprivation is a stress for the body that can lead to hormone imbalances. This can be a challenge if you have a young child who demands a lot of your time in the early evening, leading you to stay up late so that you get some time to yourself. This was a habit that I fell into when my son was young. I would stay up to midnight at times watching Netflix, enjoying the peace and quiet and time with no demands. Whilst this is fine to do occasionally, it is not great for your hormones in the long term if you do this most nights.

Exercise

Take lots of walks out in the fresh air. Aim for moderate exercise but not high intensity, as this can be another stressor to the body. Aim to engage in at least 30 minutes of moderate exercise, like brisk walking, biking, swimming, and weightlifting, five days per week.

Homeopathy

As I was over 40, I also used homeopathy to support progesterone production. Specifically, I used a New Zealand-made homeopathic remedy called Prog Aid from a company named Life Force. There are several options available, but personalised homeopathic remedies work best when tailored to the symptoms and the individual. So, if you are interested in exploring this, it is best to work with a qualified homoeopath.

Vitex/chaste tree

The herb vitex, also called chaste tree, is well-known for its hormone-regulating properties, including the ability to increase progesterone levels and lengthen the luteal phase. I have personally used it to enhance progesterone levels, but it may not be suitable for everyone. It is not something I would just try to see what happens unless you know you have low progesterone as for some people it can really extend their cycle to over 30 days. Since I am a nutritionist and not a herbalist, I am unable to provide any specific recommendations on vitex in this book. I suggest consulting a qualified naturopath or herbalist before starting to use it to make sure it is suitable for you.

Low testosterone

A factor that is often overlooked when assessing hormones for a female client with infertility is low testosterone. This is because testosterone is predominantly seen as a male hormone and as a female, it might not feel quite right when you are told you need to increase your testosterone levels.

Low testosterone can be common in females, especially women over the age of 35, as levels naturally decline from this age. I am seeing this hormone picture pop up more and more frequently with clients when I do a DUTCH test for them. It is important to be aware of what causes it and what we can do to bring our hormones back into balance.

Why is testosterone important for females?

The adrenal glands and ovaries produce testosterone, which naturally declines over the age of 35, as with the hormone progesterone. The adrenal cortex produces DHEA, which is converted by enzymes into testosterone and estradiol (E2).

As well as aging, stress and high cortisol levels can reduce levels of testosterone by lowering the production of DHEA from the adrenal glands, which results in less DHEA available to be converted into testosterone.

If you are over the age of 40 and are trying to conceive, it is recommended that you undergo testing for testosterone and DHEA-S (DHEA sulfate is the test used). If the results show low levels, you may require additional support.

Testosterone and DHEA levels play an important role in the early stages of egg development and maturity, so a deficiency may affect egg quality. In terms of fertility, testosterone is important for:

- Regulating follicle development as testosterone supports the structure of the follicles that releases the egg during ovulation.

- Helps the growth of follicles in the ovaries by stimulating the synthesis of ovarian follicle stimulating hormone (FSH) receptors.

- Increasing blood flow to the reproductive organs, which improves the production of cervical mucus.

- Helping to increase libido around ovulation time to help things along.

What are the symptoms of low testosterone?

It is common for low testosterone symptoms to be overlooked because they can overlap with HPA axis dysfunction and symptoms of low thyroid function. Here are some of the most common symptoms:

- Low energy and fatigue

- Muscle weakness

- Low bone density

- Feels the cold easy

- Difficulty losing weight

- Poor sleep

- Depressed mood

- Anxiety

- Brain fog, lack of concentration

- Hair loss

- Low libido

- Infertility.

Sex hormone binding globulin (SHBG)

Another factor to take into consideration when analysing hormones is sex hormone binding globulin (SHBG) as it is usually tested alongside testosterone and DHEA-S. SHBG is a protein that is made mostly in the liver. It binds (attaches) to sex hormones in your blood. SHBG helps to control the amount of sex hormones that are actively working in your body. [5]

SHBG plays an important role in regulating testosterone levels by transporting it throughout the body. Elevated SHBG levels decrease the levels of free testosterone available in the body. There are many factors that increase SHBG levels, such as exercise and weight loss, but the main one is stress. High cortisol levels from stress can lead to increased SHBG levels, which is another reason stress can really play havoc with our hormones and push them out of whack.

According to Dr Jolene Brighten, 'Chronic unrelenting stress doesn't give your adrenals a break. Your body keeps pumping out cortisol, plus other hormones to try to make even more cortisol. Eventually, the production of all hormones drops, including DHEA, impacting testosterone production. While this may feel like a betrayal by your body, it is actually how your body keeps you from overproducing the pro-aging hormone cortisol.' [6]

All is not lost when our testosterone and DHEA are low, as there are many natural ways to optimise levels through our diet and lifestyle. These are:

Step 1 - Nourish with nutrients

The most supportive nutrients for increasing testosterone production are zinc, magnesium, and healthy dietary fats. Let us look at each one.

Zinc

Zinc is one of those nutrients that you can easily think you have covered because you are taking a prenatal multivitamin with zinc and eating plenty of meat. However, this may not be the case!

Zinc is involved as a cofactor in over 300 enzyme functions in the body. It is also one of the trace minerals that is rapidly depleted by stress. As well as everything else going on in our lives, infertility is stress, chronic stress, so if our zinc stores become depleted, that is over 300 metabolic functions in the body that will be affected!

Zinc helps to regulate hormones and increase testosterone levels. It does this by blocking the enzyme that converts testosterone to estrogen, so more testosterone is available. Zinc rich foods are oysters, beef, lamb, pumpkin seeds, lentils, mushrooms, spinach, and avocado. Supplementing with extra zinc may be beneficial if you are not getting enough dietary zinc, have an underactive thyroid or you are under a lot of stress.

Dietary fats

The body makes testosterone, like all reproductive hormones, from dietary cholesterol. If you are not eating enough fat, or you do not absorb fat that well because of digestive issues, then the body may not have adequate cholesterol to make hormones.

Aim to have a serving of healthy fat with each meal. This may include meat fat, butter, cheese, fermented dairy, sour cream, coconut oil, meat stock, avocado, salmon, nuts, seeds and olive oil.

Consume oily fish like tuna, salmon, sardines, and mackerel two to three times a week for an excellent source of omega-3 essential fatty acids. Flaxseed oil, hemp seed oil, walnuts, and chia seeds are also good sources. You might also consider supplementing with omega-3 if you do not feel you are getting enough in your diet. Cod liver oil has the extra benefit of naturally occurring Vitamin D and A, which helps to support hormone regulation and immune balance.

Magnesium

Low magnesium levels have a connection to low testosterone levels, and supplementing with magnesium may help to restore testosterone levels to within normal ranges. Magnesium is another mineral that is depleted by stress and is a cofactor in over 300 metabolic functions of the body.

Magnesium-rich foods include almonds, cashews, seeds, bananas, avocado, brown rice, leafy green vegetables and dark chocolate.

It is challenging to get enough magnesium from food, so taking a magnesium supplement can help to lower the stress hormone cortisol, which will have a knock-on effect of increasing DHEA and testosterone levels. This is because high levels of stress and cortisol depleted DHEA levels. Magnesium also inhibits testosterone from binding to sex hormone binding globulin (SHBG) which increases free testosterone levels in the blood.

Ashwagandha

The Ayurvedic herb ashwagandha, also known as Indian ginseng or winter cherry, is one of my favourite herbs for supporting the adrenal glands. As an adaptogen, ashwagandha helps us adapt to the stress we are experiencing by lowering cortisol levels and reducing symptoms of anxiety and sleep disturbances.

Researchers have proven that ashwagandha is effective in reducing levels of cortisol. 'High concentrations of full spectrum ashwagandha root extract reduces levels of serum cortisol, which elevates in stressful conditions.'[7]

Ashwagandha is available as a tea, capsules, or powder that you can add to your smoothie.

Step 2 - Actively work to manage stress levels

Chronic stress and HPA axis dysfunction can interfere with DHEA and testosterone production, as high cortisol levels block the production of these hormones.

Therefore, engaging in stress reduction activities is crucial when attempting to decrease cortisol levels naturally. Taking supplements won't do much if you are not taking the time to look after yourself. Here are a few suggestions to include in your daily routine:

Meditation

Commit to 10 minutes a day of meditation. If you struggle to do this yourself, there are some fantastic apps available. My two favourites are *Headspace* and *Smiling Minds*.

A daily meditation practice really helps to calm the mind. At first you might feel (like I did!) that it is a waste of time and you have too many thoughts running around in your head. However, after a week or two of regular practice, it becomes easier to drop into your calm inner space.

A 2013 study discovered that 'mindfulness meditation lowers cortisol levels in the blood, suggesting that it can lower stress and may decrease the risk of diseases that arise from stress.' [8]

Take time out to breathe

When you are feeling stressed or overwhelmed, taking a minute or two to practice deep breathing can instantly help you feel calm and relaxed. Deep breathing stimulates the vagus nerve to trigger a relaxation response which calms the body and reduces cortisol levels. Close your eyes and take a slow deep breath in for the count of four, hold your breath to the count of four and exhale to the count of four. Try to do this about seven times before you open your eyes. Observe how you feel.

Gratitude journal

Keep a journal by your bed and try to think of three things you are grateful for each night and write these down. This can have a positive effect on your mindset, so it is worth taking the time to do this every day.

Yoga

Subscribe to *Yoga with Adriene* on YouTube and aim to complete a 20-minute practice at home on most days of the week. You can pick from over 10 years of her free videos to suit what you need, for example: stress, relaxing yoga, energising yoga, etc. There are other great yoga channels out there, but this is my top pick.

Sleep

I know this is difficult if you have very young children but try where possible to get plenty of sleep. It can be tempting to stay up late to take time out for yourself (I am guilty of this!) but aim to get to bed before 10.30 pm at least three days a week.

Step 3 – Schedule time to exercise

Try to do some resistance training with some weights at least three times a week, even with light dumbbells, as this can help to increase testosterone levels naturally. This can also include exercises that use your own body weight, such as squats, lunges and planks.

Short bursts of high interval training like sprints and star jump can also increase testosterone levels, but I would advise not to do anything too over strenuous, as this will stress your adrenal glands further.

My three-step strategy of nourishing with nutrients, actively working to manage stress and resistance training can help to lower the stress hormone cortisol. This will have a positive effect on increasing DHEA and testosterone levels and your energy and vitality.

DHEA supplementation

If you do research on low testosterone in females online, you may notice that many doctors are recommending DHEA supplements to boost what is naturally declining with age, especially in America. Unfortunately, we cannot access DHEA supplements in Australia and New Zealand without a prescription, so this is something you will need to discuss with your doctor if your results show you may benefit from this. If you are under the age of 35, then you hopefully should find my three-step strategy enough to boost your testosterone levels naturally. If you are over the age of 35, then DHEA supplementation may be worth exploring with your fertility doctor, as this could be one of the missing pieces of your puzzle.

High testosterone

High testosterone levels are usually connected to the condition polycystic ovary syndrome (PCOS) and are usually a sign of a dysfunction in the ovaries. With PCOS, the ovaries make a larger amount of testosterone than normal, which results in symptoms such as acne, male pattern balding, facial hair growth (hirsutism), weight gain, irregular periods and infertility.

I am not an expert on PCOS as it was never a part of my own health journey, however what I see with clients in my clinic is that insulin resistance seems to play a part.

According to Dr Jolene Brighten, 'Blood sugar dysregulation is at the crux of many hormone imbalances, with high testosterone being no exception. As insulin climbs, it can stimulate the ovaries to produce testosterone, especially with women with PCOS. While many body tissues will begin ignoring insulin signals, your ovaries are among the few organs that will continue to remain sensitive to insulin.' [9]

To help manage insulin resistance, eat a diet that is low in sugar, have a serving of healthy fat and protein with each meal and an abundance of vegetables for fibre. This will have a beneficial effect on PCOS. Here are some supplements that may also be beneficial for high testosterone and PCOS:

Myo-inositol

The nutrient myo-inositol, otherwise known as vitamin B8, is the supplement of choice for PCOS as it not only helps with blood sugar balance and insulin resistance but also the healthy function of the ovaries and improvement in egg quality. It helps to support insulin resistance by helping cells to uptake insulin. Myo-inositol is available as a supplement; however, you can easily get it from dietary sources such as nuts, beans, legumes, soy, whole grains, dried prunes, peas, almonds, and liver.

Chromium

The mineral chromium may also be beneficial as it helps cells take up insulin and regulates blood sugar levels, so is helpful for PCOS symptoms associated with insulin resistance. If you are looking to increase your chromium intake, try incorporating meat, mussels, Brazil nuts, whole grains, grapes, broccoli, and brewer's yeast into your diet.

Zinc

As mentioned earlier in this chapter, the mineral zinc is important for the whole reproductive system, so it is no surprise that it plays a role in regulating testosterone levels. Good food sources of zinc are oysters, pumpkin seeds, meat, eggs, liver, and nuts.

Magnesium

This important mineral also plays a role in blood sugar regulation and insulin sensitivity alongside chromium. Good food sources are leafy green, vegetables, avocados, nuts, seeds, bananas, legumes and dark chocolate.

Promoting healthy ovulation

Delayed or absent ovulation can happen to most women from time to time. It sure did with me. However, if it happens regularly, then it is likely to be connected to a hormone imbalance which can be driven by multiple factors.

Some of the most common factors are stress, poor sleep, over-exercising, a low-calorie diet, low body weight, poor diet, nutritional deficiencies, thyroid issues, thyroid medications, an autoimmune condition, adrenal issues, PCOS, blood sugar dysregulation, poor gut health and infections. Investigating all these areas holistically with your health practitioner is a good idea to get to the root cause of what is causing the imbalance.

Normal ovulation can occur anytime from days 14 - 21. If ovulation occurs later than day 21, the quality of the egg may not be that viable and can reduce the chances of conceiving that cycle.

One of the most influential ways to promote regular ovulation is through nutrition, as we need to be supplying our bodies with the nutrient building blocks to synthesise and regulate hormones daily. In chapter three, I discussed how eating a clean, nourishing whole food diet is the best place to start when optimising fertility.

Choose food made lovingly from scratch and limit refined sugar and processed carbohydrates, even if they are gluten-free ones. We should strive to include in our diet five to eight servings of fresh fruits and vegetables, gluten-free whole grains, moderate organic meats, poultry, fish, organic dairy, nuts, seeds, legumes, fermented foods, and healthy fats.

The most important nutrients for ovulation are the B-complex vitamins especially folate, vitamin B6 and B12, plus vitamin D, iron, and essential fatty acids. It is important to make sure you are not deficient in any of these nutrients as vitamin and mineral deficiencies can lead to delayed ovulation.

Taking a quality preconception multivitamin with activated B vitamins is important to ensure you are getting a top up of all the nutrients you need. Both mum and dad to be should take a preconception multivitamin, not just the female. You can get both male and female specific preconception multivitamins.

Fibroids

It is common for females over the age of 35 to have fibroids, and you may not be aware that you have one, which was the case with me.

Fibroids are non-cancerous growths that form within the walls of the uterus. About 7 out of 10 women can have fibroids by age 50. They can vary in size, ranging from the size of a pea to as large as a melon and can form in any part of the uterus.

It is not known exactly how fibroids develop, however, there appears to be a connection with estrogen dominance. High levels of estrogen are thought to encourage the growth of fibroids, which may explain why they are more common in females over age 35.

According to Jean Hailes, infertility is not a common problem for women with fibroids as less than 3% of women have fertility problems because of fibroids. Depending on the size and position, fibroids may interfere with the implantation of the embryo into the uterus, increase the risk of miscarriage and impact the progress of labour.' [10]

I did not know that I had a fibroid until I had a scan at my fertility clinic when they were doing all the checks and tests that they do with new clients. It was situated at the top of my uterus in the centre. My fertility doctor assured me that fibroids are very common and should not hinder my ability to conceive. Since I experienced no pain and had regular periods, I wasn't really concerned about the fibroid.

In 2012, when I miscarried at six and a half weeks, I had to have a scan after a D & C procedure to check that the baby had been removed. The lady performing the scan pointed out my fibroid again. In fact, every scan I ever had in relation to fertility and pregnancy, my fibroid was pointed out to me, even during my 12- and 20-week scans with my daughter. There was the baby and there was the fibroid! However, it remained small and did not grow, and the scans showed it to be relatively harmless, which brought me some relief. It just never went away.

I wonder if the fibroid had also been present when I gave birth to my son in 2008 and was the reason I had a postpartum haemorrhage. I also had excess bleeding after my D & C and a postpartum haemorrhage with my daughter as well, even though she was a c-section baby. Although I will never know, I wonder if there is a connection there.

Natural treatments to reduce fibroids

I tried several natural remedies to reduce my fibroid over the years, but when you can't see what is going on inside you; it is hard to monitor if what you are taking is actually working. I discovered through research that fibroids are often caused by estrogen dominance. Therefore, I regularly took the supplement DIM and consumed broccoli, and broccoli sprouts to aid in the elimination of excess estrogen through the liver.

I also discovered that there is a correlation between fibroids and low levels of vitamin D, so I used muscle testing to determine if I needed to take vitamin D. It surprised me to find that I needed to take quite large doses of it daily. Muscle testing is a useful tool when you want a quick answer on whether you need to take a particular supplement at that moment in time. I sought confirmation by having my vitamin D tested, which I discovered was low, so I took 5,000 iu per day for a month to get my levels up. As a maintenance, I took 2,000 iu per day, and I hoped that this was one reason my fibroid didn't grow any bigger.

In 2019, a double-blind prospective clinical trial was performed on 69 patients with uterine fibroids who also had vitamin D deficiency. After the women in the trial began taking vitamin D supplementation, the researchers observed a significant reduction in the size of the fibroids. The study concluded that the administration of vitamin D may reduce the size of fibroids. [11]

If you suspect that a uterine fibroid is affecting your fertility, I suggest getting your vitamin D levels checked and taking a daily dose of 2,000 iu, particularly during winter when sun exposure is limited.

Next steps

In summary, if you suspect you may have a hormone imbalance such as estrogen dominance or low progesterone, I recommend increasing foods that help to support the detoxification of estrogen, such as foods rich in sulforaphane (broccoli and broccoli sprouts) and lightly cooked brassica vegetables. You should also review what xenoestrogens you may be exposed to in your environment, reduce the use of plastic containers, and change your cosmetics if necessary.

You may also need to look at your stress levels and how you can find more relaxation and balance in your life, as high amounts of stress can lead to HPA axis dysfunction, which could be affecting progesterone levels.

If you regularly experience a few digestive issues, then it would be worth trying to resolve these by focusing on the steps mentioned in the gut health chapter, such as increasing water intake, probiotic and prebiotic foods, and foods rich in polyphenols. If your gut issues do not resolve by taking these actions, you may wish to work with a practitioner like myself to investigate further the root cause of your symptoms. Maybe you have food intolerances aggravating your symptoms or a bacterial or fungal overgrowth that needs attention.

Don't guess, test

If there is ever a time that we should be testing (where possible and affordable) and not guessing what is happening with our hormones, is with unexplained infertility. A good example of this is my client who has been treating herself for estrogen dominance by taking the supplement DIM, which helps the body detox excess estrogens. She thought that she had estrogen dominance as she has endometriosis and fibroids, and these conditions can in many cases be linked to estrogen dominance but not in every case.

I organised a DUTCH test for her, and her results were very interesting. She actually had very low estrogen that was tanking out at the bottom of the reference range. Without adequate estrogen the lining of the uterus is not a healthy thickness for a fertilised egg to implant and ovulation can also be impaired.

Her estrogen metabolism was mainly down the 2 OH (the good) pathway so there was no sign of any issues with her estrogen detoxification, maybe due to the DIM. Testosterone and DHEA levels were very low as well and progesterone was within normal range. The stress hormone cortisol was very high which was probably contributing to low DHEA and therefore the low testosterone and estrogen.

The point is if you work with a qualified practitioner to get testing done with say the DUTCH test, you will get to the problem sooner and can work on balancing your hormones with appropriate treatment strategies that are not going to cause a further imbalance. I find it interesting that each of my clients have a completely unique hormone profile from completing the DUTCH test, highlighting that we are all individuals, and one size does not fit all.

DUTCH testing

We are very fortunate these days to be able to investigate hormones on a deeper level with a dried urine test called the DUTCH test. With the DUTCH test, you can get a comprehensive hormone analysis that includes hormone metabolites, organic acids, methylation, and oxidative stress markers. It is especially useful for investigating adrenal function, estrogen and progesterone balance, androgen deficiency or excess, and whether the metabolism of hormones is sluggish or overactive.

I often organise a DUTCH test for my clients, and I am trained to interpret the results, which can seem quite complex when you first look at it as there is so much valuable information. The DUTCH test is a great way to investigate what is really happening with your hormones, as it not only provides information on free hormones but downstream metabolites as well, which tells us how the hormones are functioning.

Chapter Six

Fertility over 40

T rying to get pregnant when you are over 40 is a challenge, as the odds are firmly stacked against you. However, it is still a possibility, so there is always hope.

For me, it was a self-development project. I was fortunate enough to conceive and give birth to my miracle baby at age 44, but I worked really hard for it for a very long time. For over 10 years, I made a lot of sacrifices on my journey to get pregnant. I avoided certain foods in case I was pregnant, cut out caffeine and alcohol, invested in supplements that may be helpful when the money was needed elsewhere, and avoided high intensity exercise, which was something I loved the most.

When I was told my anti-mullerian hormone (AMH) was low at age 39 and that my chances of getting pregnant via IVF were quite slim, this motivated me to become the healthiest version of myself that I could be. When my IVF pregnancy ended in a miscarriage at age 41 and I was told my only hope was to use a donor as my eggs were too old, my instinct told me that was not true. I believed that I needed to keep going, keep trying, keep striving to become the healthiest version of myself I could be.

I continued to strive for optimal health and by the time I conceived my miracle daughter naturally at age 43, I was the healthiest I had been in my entire life. My gut symptoms and skin rashes were gone, and my asthma was under control. I guess I was fortunate to be a nutritionist and have access to practitioner research, resources and supplements that many don't have access to. This is why it is now time for me to use this knowledge to benefit others.

One of the biggest frustrations we are told when we are trying to conceive is that it is a "numbers game" and that our miscarriage or failed IVF cycle was because of a genetically bad egg and that we just need to keep trying month after month until we are successful. This is not true! We can't expect to do the same thing over and over again and expect a different outcome. We need to look at why this is happening and what we can build on with our diet and lifestyle to move forward. Even if you just take one thing to improve on each month, for example reducing sugar or taking that probiotic, to keep yourself moving in the right direction.

I was listening to a fertility webinar for practitioners last year and Angela Hywood, a renowned fertility naturopath in Australia, quoted, "If you conceive and give birth to a healthy baby in your forties, you have the potential to live to 100". I have to agree with this. If you are looking to get pregnant in your forties, your health needs to be the best it can be and then some. Try not to waste any time trying different supplements just because you heard about it in a forum. Everyone is different and what works for some may not be what you need.

Whether you are new to the fertility journey or experiencing challenges, I advise taking a break from trying to conceive and dedicating three to four months to a preconception care program for both partners to enhance your overall health. Three months is the average time it takes for eggs to mature and for new sperm to be produced. I know it is hard when you feel like time is running out, but you really need to take a break from trying to conceive during this time as you want to make sure your eggs are healthy ones, a reflection of your hard work during the three months you spent getting your health on track.

Another thing that is hard to accept but is a reality when trying to conceive over the age of 40 is that in most cases, you will need to take supplements, and likely more than one. There is unfortunately not a quick fix or magic bullet, and if you are over 40, you may well have a few nutritional deficiencies or hormone imbalances that need addressing. Or you might have inflammation or a gut issue that needs some attention. This is just the reality of being an older mum. It takes a huge amount of physical effort and resources to conceive, carry to term, deliver a healthy baby, and then breastfeed in your 40s (if you are able to). At the point of writing this, I am 46 and I have a very active 21-month-old. I feel that my resources have been drained and I am very depleted. My health is not as great as it was before I was pregnant, and I look and feel much older. That's the reality of being a mum in your 40s. It is exhausting, so your body needs to be really ready for it.

Take advantage of the four-month preconception period to nourish your body with fertility-enhancing nutrients, resolve gut issues, reduce inflammation, balance hormones, and optimise the function of your reproductive organs. Treat this time as a wellbeing holiday and try not to worry about getting pregnant. This may be all you need. Try not to waste time playing the numbers game, or you may run out of time.

What are the chances of getting pregnant over the age of 40?

It is a reality that fertility declines dramatically over the age of 40. This is because of the decrease in the number of eggs that remain in the ovaries, which reduces the chances of conceiving each month. Maintaining a pregnancy can also be a challenge as the incidence of miscarriage increases with age.

According to the American Society of Reproductive Medicine, by age 40, a woman's chance of conceiving is less than 5% per cycle, so fewer than 5 out of every 100 are expected to be successful each month. [1]

The US Centre for Disease Control and Prevention (CDC) quote that 30% of women between the ages of 40 and 44 experience infertility. The reduction in female fertility after age 40 happens because of a natural age-related decline in egg quality and quantity. As women get older, more of their eggs have abnormal numbers of chromosomes, which increases the chance of miscarriage. When eggs have genetic abnormalities, even if they are fertilised, there is a high chance that the pregnancy won't be able to continue. By age 40, less than 50% of women's eggs are genetically normal. Also, 34% of pregnancies in women between the age of 40–44 end in miscarriage and this increases to 53% for women over the age of 45. [2]

I came across some interesting statistics from an article published online by the Virginia Physicians for Women. Their article highlights that when girls are born, their ovaries contain the total number of eggs they will ever have, which is around one million. The numbers decline with age and most women lose about 30 immature eggs a day! This means that by the time a woman reaches puberty, her ovaries contain 300,000 eggs and by the age of 30, she is down to 100,000 eggs. It is estimated that by age 40, women only have about 20,000 eggs remaining. [3]

Another factor to consider is that after age 40, you have a higher chance of being diagnosed with other age-related conditions that may affect fertility. Examples of this are blood sugar issues, insulin resistance, weight gain, high blood pressure, thyroid issues and autoimmune conditions.

This all sounds a bit doom and gloom if you are currently trying to conceive and you are over the age of 40, but it doesn't mean there isn't a reason to be hopeful. Despite the odds being stacked against me, I conceived naturally at age 43 after 10 years of secondary infertility and recurrent pregnancy loss, and I gave birth at age 44 to a healthy baby girl.

Improving egg quality

If you are trying to conceive over the age of 40, your focus needs to be on improving the quality of the remaining eggs you have available in your ovaries.

Optimal ovarian health is required for an egg to develop from its immature state to one that is ready for ovulation and capable of being fertilised, a process that takes around three months. Egg development requires a great deal of cellular energy and as women age, the ovaries become less efficient at meeting the demands of the growing egg. This affects egg quality and increases the chances of genetic errors occurring.

Coenzyme Q10

To improve egg quality, an essential nutrient to take as a supplement is coenzyme Q10 in the form of ubiquinol, its most bioavailable and absorbable form.

Coenzyme Q10 is a powerful antioxidant that helps to protect eggs from free radical damage. It is an essential nutrient for fertility over the age of 40 and for mitochondrial health. Taking coenzyme Q10 for about three months before trying to conceive may help to improve egg quality and increase your chances of pregnancy and favourable IVF outcomes. A 2018 study investigated the effects of coenzyme Q10 on ovarian response and embryo quality in women with poor ovarian response. 'Women in the coenzyme Q10 group had an increased number of retrieved oocytes, higher fertilisation rates, and higher quality embryos.' [4]

Coenzyme Q10 is also important for supporting the health of the mitochondria, which is our energy powerhouse at the centre of each cell in our body. Therefore, it is essential to prioritise mitochondrial health when trying to conceive after the age of 40.

What are the mitochondria?

The mitochondria, found at the centre of every cell in our body, is essentially our battery power, our energy source. They produce cellular energy from the food that we eat by breaking down glucose into adenosine triphosphate (ATP), the cell's main energy molecule that is used to fuel various other cellular processes. So, you can understand the critical role of mitochondria in our function and survival.

If mitochondrial energy production is compromised, it can cause weakness, fatigue, can accelerate aging, and is linked to infertility, especially in women over the age of 35.

According to Lee Know 'The reason the mitochondria are so important for fertility is that each oocyte contains about 100,000 mitochondria and defective or dysfunctional mitochondria are a key contributor to infertility in women over the age of 35.' [5] After fertilisation, the zygote goes through rapid cell division, which requires a huge amount of cellular energy. If there is not enough cellular energy to separate chromosomes during cell division, this can lead to chromosomal abnormalities such as down's syndrome. This is one of the primary reasons older women have a higher chance of giving birth to babies with birth defects. 'Early embryo and implantation potential has been correlated with mitochondrial function and activity.' [6]

Coenzyme Q10 is an important compound that plays an essential role in mitochondria function and our ability to produce coenzyme Q10 naturally declines with age. As our aging bodies naturally produce less and less coenzyme Q10, we naturally produce less and less cellular energy, which is essential for reproductive function. This is why low levels of coenzyme Q10 can contribute to infertility. If the body does not produce enough coenzyme Q10, it may compromise the quality of the female egg. Additionally, if fertilisation occurs, the fertilised egg may not generate enough cellular energy to divide properly, resulting in chromosomal abnormalities and miscarriage.

Coenzyme Q10 not only plays a key role in protecting DNA at the cellular level and improving egg health in women, but also sperm health in men. As an antioxidant, it helps to protect both the egg and sperm from oxidative stress and harmful free radical damage.

Mitochondrial function declines from around age 35. 'In patients over 38 years of age, most of the luteal granulosa cells from preovulatory follicles exhibit an abnormal mitochondrial morphology and reduced expression of crucial antioxidant enzymes compared to women younger than 32 years of age.' [7]

What is coenzyme Q10 and where do we get it from?

Coenzyme Q10 is a vitamin-like compound that we can make in our bodies and obtain through food. It naturally declines with age. The best food sources are beef, lamb, pork, organ meat, and oily fish such as salmon, mackerel, and sardines. Plant sources such as whole grains, green leafy vegetables, spinach, kale, broccoli, and nuts are also a source of coenzyme Q10, but they have much lower levels. Vegans and vegetarians are at a greater risk of a deficiency, as they don't consume the richer animal sources. When we eat meat, we consume all the benefits from the animal, including their mitochondria.

There is research that supports supplementing with coenzyme Q10 for any female over the age of 35 who is trying to conceive. Coenzyme Q10 can also provide valuable support for anyone undergoing fertility treatments such as IVF. The recommendation is for both the male and female to take ubiquinol at least three months prior to the procedure.

According to Rebecca Fett in her book *It starts with the Egg*, supplementing with 200 - 600 mg per day of coenzyme Q10 as ubiquinol is one of the best ways to improve egg quality. 'Given everything we know about how coenzyme Q10 increases energy production in the mitochondria, how important this energy production is for egg and embryo development and the positive results from clinical studies to date, the current evidence suggests that adding a ubiquinol supplement is one of the best ways to improve egg quality' [8]

How else can we support our mitochondria and, therefore, our egg quality?

To maintain healthy mitochondria, it is important to eat a diet high in antioxidants that can neutralise free radicals and protect against oxidative stress. Eating a variety of brightly coloured fruits and vegetables is a great way to supply the body with a rich source of antioxidants. Fruits such as blueberries, strawberries, raspberries, and Goji berries are excellent sources. Also, leafy green vegetables like kale and spinach, red cabbage, red grapes, and dark chocolate.

Magnesium is another nutrient that is important for ATP cellular energy production in the mitochondria as well as the B-complex vitamins, omega-3 and alpha lipoic acid.

Alpha lipoic acid (ALA)

In this section, I will give you more details about alpha lipoic acid (ALA), which might be new to you. We covered magnesium, omega-3, and B vitamins in chapter three. Alpha lipoic acid is not something that is necessary for everyone to take while trying to conceive, however can be beneficial for mitochondrial support if you are trying to conceive over the age of 40.

Alpha lipoic acid is a compound that is made in the mitochondria of all body cells and has a role in converting nutrients into cellular energy. It is also a powerful antioxidant that protects the mitochondria from age related oxidative damage, which helps to improve the function of the mitochondria.

A study published in the *Journal of Fertility and Sterility* found that supplementing with 400 mg of alpha lipoic acid for 60–90 days increased the number of mature good quality eggs and embryos a woman produced. Pregnancy rates were also higher for women who took alpha lipoic acid supplements compared to the control group, though the difference didn't reach a statistically significant level. [9]

Not forgetting the men, in a 2015 study, men taking 600 mg per day of alpha lipoic acid experienced improved sperm count and motility. [10]

Alpha lipoic acid can therefore be beneficial for both male and female fertility, especially if you are trying to conceive over the age of 40. Supporting your mitochondrial health is critical for improving egg and sperm quality and the prevention of miscarriage.

Along with supplements, you can also boost your intake of alpha lipoic acid by consuming nutrient-dense foods. Red meat, liver, carrots, beetroot, spinach, Brussel sprouts, broccoli, potatoes, and brewer's yeast are all good options.

Boron

Boron is an underrated mineral that is important for hormone balance and fertility over the age of 40. It was a supplement that I started taking about three months before I got pregnant naturally at age 43 after 10 years of secondary infertility and recurrent pregnancy loss. Since I made other changes at the same time, I didn't fully appreciate the importance of boron until a similar situation occurred with one of my clients. After three months of working with me to support her nutrition, my client discovered she was pregnant at age 43 after experiencing multiple pregnancy losses. She made other changes to her diet, lifestyle, and supplement regime over those three months, so it is unclear if boron played a part in her getting pregnant, but we would like to think so. The knowledge that it has happened twice, though, has made me pay some more attention to this underrated mineral.

I started taking boron about three months before I conceived at age 43. The reason I started taking it was because I felt I was entering the beginning stages of perimenopause, and my hormones were out of balance. After doing some research on perimenopause, I felt it would be useful to try. As a practitioner who worked in a health shop, I would often research supplements and experiment on myself to see what happens and pass on any lessons to my clients. I had a lot going on at the time, so I didn't really notice a big difference when I took it, but that's usually the case with hormone supporting supplements. The changes are often subtle, and it can take a few months to notice the benefit.

What is boron and how does it help with hormone balance?

Boron is an important trace mineral that is not talked about that often, especially in terms of fertility. This may be because there is a lack of knowledge about the importance of boron, but also there is limited clinical research about the mineral and its uses. There still seems to be lots to learn about this mineral.

If you eat plenty of fruit, vegetables, nuts, and legumes in theory, you should be getting enough boron from food. However, there are certainly times in our lives when we could do with supplementing with some extra boron. One of those times would be during perimenopause, menopause, or if you are trying to conceive and you are over the age of 40. This is because boron can increase estrogen and testosterone levels in women, and if you are perimenopausal or trying to conceive over 40, these are the hormones that can start to get erratic and for many women are on a natural decline. Estrogen and testosterone are important not only for egg quality but also for healthy ovulation, healthy libido, and a sense of wellbeing.

When I had IVF at age 41, I completed the long cycle procedure in which the fertility clinic manages your complete cycle using various drugs and hormones. I distinctly remember having to take a drug that suppressed the production of estrogen for about a week; I think it was to get the timing of my cycle within their schedule. So, for about a week I was surviving on little or no estrogen and my goodness, I felt terrible. My face seemed puffy and had aged within a week, and I was having hot flushes at night. I remember a colleague at work telling me that there was something different about me and that I looked older. That is the effect of low estrogen. I felt older, like I had lost my spark.

Not only does boron play a crucial role in the synthesis of estradiol (E2) and testosterone, but it also plays a role in maintaining a healthy balance of other reproductive hormones. 'Numerous studies indicate that boron intake affects the presence or function of hormones, including vitamin D, estrogen, thyroid hormone, insulin, and progesterone.' [11]

Enhancing dietary boron intake can have many benefits, including increased fertility, vitality, and the reduction of perimenopausal symptoms and PMS, which are the consequence of hormones that are out of balance. 'In animal studies, boron depletion is linked to fertility problems and birth defects, which suggests that boron can play a role in healthy reproduction and fetus development.' [12]

Boron has many beneficial functions besides fertility. This mighty trace mineral is also:

- Essential for bone health and metabolism as it helps the body produce and utilise vitamin D, calcium, and magnesium

- Involved in regulating estrogen and testosterone

- Anti-inflammatory, so helpful for any chronic inflammation

- Supportive of brain health and cognitive performance

- A nutrient that increases glutathione levels, the body's main antioxidant. It helps to protect against oxidative stress

- Anti-fungal. It may help to reduce yeast infections, as boron (as boric acid) is an active ingredient in tablets used to treat yeast infections in women. This means that taking boron as a supplement may help to treat common yeast infections such as candida albicans

Food Sources of boron

You may think, wow, this boron mineral sounds amazing. What do I need to eat to increase my boron levels? As mentioned earlier in this chapter, if you eat well and eat a variety of fruits, vegetables, nuts, and legumes, you should be getting enough boron in your diet. Foods that are rich in boron are avocados, apples, pears, oranges, grapes, grapes, leafy greens, peanuts, pecans, red kidney beans and lentils.

At the time of writing this, there is not a set adequate intake level for boron, despite the many studies showing the beneficial effects of boron. Instead, the United States Institute of Medicine Food and Nutrition Board has set a tolerable upper intake level of 20 mg/d for adults, which includes pregnancy and breastfeeding. Research suggests that 3–5 mg a day is considered an optimal range, and many supplements on the market are in 3 mg doses.

According to Jillian Levy 'the risks of consuming this mineral are thought to be minimal, especially from natural food sources. It is widely recognised as being very safe for consumption in both humans and animals. The only caution would be with people with hormone sensitive conditions like breast or prostate cancer, endometriosis or uterine fibroids since supplementing with boron can increase estrogen levels.' [13]

I think we will hear more about the benefits of boron as more research comes into light. Boron's anti-inflammatory, antioxidant, hormone balancing, and mineral metabolism properties make it a vital part of improving fertility in all females, but especially females over the age of 40. Forrest Nielsen and Susan Meacham suggest that boron intakes above 1 mg/day could help people live "longer and better." [14] We can do this simply by eating more fruits, vegetables, nuts, and pulses. I am up for that.

Chapter summary

If you are trying to get pregnant over the age of 40, your health needs to be the best it can be and then some. Even with a healthy diet, you are likely to need to take a few supplements.

Three months is the average time it takes for eggs to mature and new sperm to be produced. This highlights the importance of a three-month preconception health care plan for optimising fertility and egg quality.

Coenzyme Q10 is important for egg quality and supporting mitochondrial health, which is important for fertility over the age of 40. The preferred choice of coenzyme Q10 supplement is as ubiquinol. The antioxidant alpha lipoic acid can provide further support by protecting the mitochondria from age related oxidative damage.

Boron is an important trace mineral for hormone balance and shows potential as a support for improved fertility outcomes over the age of 40.

Chapter Seven

Stress

Anyone who has been on a journey trying to conceive will have been told at some stage by well-meaning friends and relatives to "just relax and stop stressing" and it will more likely happen. We have all heard stories of someone we know who, after seven failed IVF procedures, gave up trying to conceive to focus on a new career only to get pregnant naturally, or a friend who, after years of infertility, conceived while on a relaxing holiday. So, we understand that stress affects us, but why is this? What happens in the body when we are under pressure and how does this really affect fertility? Understanding this can be a real "ah-ha" moment and can help motivate you to look at how stress can be affecting you.

It is all about our hormones

Without a healthy balance of hormones, getting pregnant or staying pregnant can be a challenge. It is also very hard for anyone to have a healthy balance of hormones unless your life is in balance. For optimal hormonal health, we need to balance all areas of our lives, whether physical, emotional or spiritual. These include:

- Work and a sense of purpose

- Family and relationships

- Exercise - not too much or not too little

- Healthy diet

- Sleep, relaxation, and me-time

- Having fun

- Gut health, allergies, and infections

- Nutritional deficiencies

- Physical alignment and pain

- Space in your life for a baby

It is hard not to feel stressed when you are experiencing infertility. It is an emotional rollercoaster filled with hope at the start of your cycle and very often crushing disappointment at the end of your monthly cycle if your period shows up. Then there will be a few days of sadness until you bounce back and start all over again with the next cycle. You have to put on a smile and hope that this next cycle is the one.

The unfortunate reality about stress is that it messes with every single hormone, especially progesterone, the important hormone for maintaining a pregnancy.

The corpus luteum of the ovary produces progesterone from approximately day 14–28 of your cycle. As well as this, a percentage of progesterone is also produced by the adrenal glands that regulate the stress response. This means that if you are under a lot of stress, then your adrenal glands may have shut down your production of progesterone in favour of stress hormones such as cortisol and adrenaline. I really believe this was a huge factor in my fertility journey and is likely to be the case with many women in this day and age. Stress literally shuts down our reproductive system, since getting pregnant is not considered essential for our survival, unlike our heart and circulation.

The problem is that many women experiencing infertility are stuck in a permanent state of high alert and their bodies remain in survival mode long term, which is not the ideal environment to conceive and maintain a healthy pregnancy.

During my 10-year journey with secondary infertility, I was studying, raising a child, working part time in a health shop, and starting up my clinic as a nutritionist. This was, at the same time as dealing with the emotional difficulties of infertility. I thought I was doing all the right things to keep my hormones in balance, but obviously, I wasn't. It was only when I quit working in the health shop in 2018 to focus purely on my clinic work, I discovered I was pregnant three weeks later at age 43. Maybe it was because I reduced my stress levels, or maybe I had finally made space in my life to have time to look after a baby. These are all important factors that play a part in having a healthy balance of hormones.

Stress also leads to an increase in the production of the stress hormone cortisol from the adrenal glands, which inhibits GnRH (gonadotropin-releasing hormone). The role of GnRH is to trigger the pituitary gland to secrete luteinising hormone (LH) and follicle-stimulating hormone (FSH), so if stress suppresses these hormones, ovulation may not occur. In men, stress can have a negative effect on sperm health.

Chronic stress can lead to HPA axis dysfunction, which can down regulate your thyroid gland and lead to an underactive thyroid. Having thyroid issues can negatively affect your fertility as well as your energy levels and sense of wellbeing. I will cover more on thyroid dysfunction in the next chapter.

Stress is more than just being busy. If you have an injury, infection, gut issue, or food intolerance that is causing inflammation and uncomfortable symptoms, this is stressful for your body as well. These situations can weaken the immune system and can become a form of stress that affects your whole glandular system.

So, if you are on the infertility rollercoaster, then maybe it is time to take stock and consider what is causing you the most stress in your life, whether it is emotional or physical, and what action you can take to reduce this.

HPA axis dysfunction (adrenal fatigue)

As discussed in chapter 5, the hypothalamus, pituitary, and adrenal glands make up the HPA axis, which regulates our adaptive response to stress. HPA axis dysfunction (or adrenal fatigue, which is otherwise known) is when our adrenal glands function below optimal levels, usually because of prolonged chronic stress. The adrenal glands are located on top of the kidneys and regulate our stress response by producing stress hormones such as cortisol and adrenaline in response to stress. Long-term stress can lead to the depletion of the adrenal glands and can cause imbalances in the production of cortisol. When the body is in an alert stressed state, non-essential functions that are not important for immediate survival, such as the digestive system, reproduction system, and thyroid, start to slow down and down regulate. This can make it a challenge to keep our reproductive hormones in a healthy balance.

'The hypothalamic-pituitary-adrenal (HPA) axis, when activated by stress, exerts an inhibitory effect on the female reproductive system. Corticotrophin-releasing hormone (CRH) inhibits hypothalamic gonadotropin-releasing hormone (GnRH), and glucocorticoids inhibit pituitary luteinizing hormone and ovarian estrogen and progesterone secretion.' [1]

Poor egg quality is associated with HPA dysfunction because high levels of cortisol, and the inhibition of LH, affects follicular development and oocyte quality. 'Follicular fluid from follicles whose oocytes were not fertilised had levels of cortisol significantly higher than levels in follicular fluid from follicles containing successfully fertilised oocytes. This suggests that high levels of glucocorticoids negatively influence the ability of an oocyte to become fertilised.' [2] Here are some of the most common symptoms of HPA axis dysfunction:

- Exhaustion and fatigue

- Waking up unrefreshed after a long sleep

- Brain fog, concentration issues

- 3 pm energy crash

- Craving sugar, coffee, or salt

- Tired in the evenings but gets second wind after 10 pm and stays up late

- Hormone imbalances, such as low progesterone and testosterone

- Thyroid dysfunction

- Infertility and recurrent miscarriage

- Weight gain around the middle

- Blood sugar issues

Nutrients to support the adrenal glands

The two most supportive nutrients for the adrenal glands are vitamin C and vitamin B5 (pantothenic acid). The adrenal glands need both vitamin B5 and vitamin C to function optimally and produce adrenal hormones.

Vitamin B5 (pantothenic acid)

Vitamin B5, also known as pantothenic acid, enhances adrenal gland function. It is involved in the production of adrenal hormones that help to reduce stress and plays a key role in energy metabolism. Vitamin B5 is known as the "anti-stress hormone" and we use up more of it when we are experiencing periods of stress. A deficiency can contribute to adrenal dysfunction.

Many foods contain vitamin B5, and our gut bacteria also manufactures it in the colon, so a deficiency is not that common. However, people who have diets high in refined processed foods and have poor gut health are more likely to be deficient. Some of the best food choices of vitamin B5 are brewers' yeast, liver, egg yolks, fish, chicken, lentils, whole grains, cheese, peanuts, cashew nuts, dried beans, green peas, cauliflower, mushrooms, and avocados. Some of the deficiency signs to be aware of are:

- Fatigue

- Allergies

- Poor digestion, abdominal cramps

- Blood sugar issues

- Skin problems

- Tingling in hands and feet

- Recurring upper respiratory symptoms

Supplementation with vitamin B5 can be helpful if fatigue is an issue. If you are supplementing with a single B vitamin, it is also important to take a separate B-complex containing all the B group vitamins, preferably in an activated form in case of methylation issues. This is because the B-complex vitamins work synergistically as a family and an excess of one B vitamin over the long term can cause deficiencies in others.

Vitamin C

Vitamin C increases adrenal function as it is involved in the production of adrenal hormones. The adrenal glands store and utilise vitamin C, so when the body is under prolonged stress, vitamin C levels in the adrenal glands can become depleted. Vitamin C is therefore an essential nutrient to optimise with food and supplements daily if you are experiencing periods of prolonged stress, especially as vitamin C is a water-soluble vitamin that is easily excreted from the body.

Vitamin C is also an important nutrient for supporting ovarian function. It helps to promote ovulation and improves progesterone levels by lengthening the luteal phase. Here are some signs of vitamin C deficiency:

- Poor immunity

- Slow wound healing

- Bleeding gums

- Easy bruising

- Fatigue

- Dandruff

- Rough skin

Some of the best sources of vitamin C are oranges, lemons, limes, tangerines, grape-fruit, rose hips, acerola berries, strawberries, red and green peppers, broccoli, potatoes, tomatoes, asparagus, and Brussel sprouts.

I like to supplement with around 1,000 mg a day of liposomal vitamin C, which comes in a liquid form. The liposomal technology enhances absorption by encasing the vitamin C in a liposome, which is a microscopic lipid coating that carries the nutrient directly into the cells.

Magnesium

In times of stress, magnesium is the mineral supplement of choice, as it is known as the relaxing mineral. Magnesium is a very important macro (major) mineral that we require daily in quite substantial amounts, which is around 400 mg a day. Yet it is one of the most common nutritional deficiencies in the world and a deficiency of magnesium can lead to several health complaints, especially related to stress, sleep problems, cramps and energy levels.

Magnesium is involved in over 300 metabolic and enzymatic functions in the body. This means if you are deficient in magnesium, you essentially have around 300 metabolic functions that are not working efficiently. This ultimately leads to dysfunction, as the body struggles to maintain homeostasis (a healthy balance) without this important mineral.

When we are under stress, our metabolic need for magnesium increases, resulting in the rapid depletion of our magnesium stores. Magnesium is a critical mineral for adrenal function as it is not only depleted by stress, but it is also the key nutrient that helps us deal with stress. When we are deficient in magnesium, symptoms like anxiety, sleep issues, and even high blood pressure emerge. Here are some common signs that you are deficient in magnesium:

- Frequent headaches and migraines (also consider dehydration)

- Muscle cramps and twitches (e.g. eyelids), restless legs

- Premenstrual tension, cramps, infertility, menopausal issues

- Anxiety, tension, inability to relax, low tolerance to stress

- Insomnia and difficulty falling asleep

- Asthma

- High blood pressure

- Low energy and fatigue

- Hypoglycaemia and blood sugar issues

- Chronic constipation

- Heart palpitations, irregular heartbeat.

If you crave dark chocolate, this is also a sign that you are deficient in magnesium, as dark chocolate is a rich source of magnesium.

So why are we so deficient in magnesium?

The soils in New Zealand (and possibly worldwide) lack magnesium, as well as other important minerals like selenium and iodine. Additionally, food processing results in an 80% loss of magnesium.

The modern diet lacks sufficient consumption of foods that are good sources of magnesium, such as nuts, seeds, and leafy greens. Also, stress, excess sugar intake, alcohol and many common medications such as corticosteroids and the oral contraceptive pill further deplete magnesium levels. Many people also have gastrointestinal diseases, such as coeliac disease or inflammatory bowel disease, which can affect the absorption of minerals.

Good food sources of magnesium are almonds, Brazil nuts, pumpkin seeds, sunflower seeds, leafy greens (kale, spinach), bananas, chickpeas, beans, shrimp, and raw cacao.

If you eat a lot of these foods and still have some magnesium deficiency symptoms, you may benefit from an additional magnesium glycinate supplement, as this is the better absorbed form of magnesium. Magnesium glycinate is my preferred form of magnesium, as it is great for sensitive individuals. Where possible, avoid supplements with magnesium oxide as absorption is very low, so it is not great at getting your magnesium levels up, but it does, however, work as a laxative for constipation.

Epsom salts baths

One of my favourite stress management tools is to relax in a bath with Epsom salts a few times a week. The minerals magnesium and sulfate make up Epsom salts and the skin directly absorbs them. Magnesium calms the nervous system and muscles, so is very good as a de-stress at the end of a tough day. A 10–15-minute bath with Epsom salt also helps draw out toxins from the skin, aiding in natural detoxification.

To take a bath with Epsom salts, dissolve 250g (1 cup) into a warm bath (not too hot) and soak for 10 - 15 minutes. Epsom salts are available in pharmacies, health shops, and supermarkets and cost around $3 for a 500g bag. I recommend drinking some water before your Epsom salt bath, as you can get a little thirsty.

Adrenal glandular

During my fertility journey, I supported my adrenals daily with an adrenal glandular supplement, which I felt made a vast difference to my energy levels and feeling of wellbeing. Adrenal glandular supplements can be a useful support for the adrenals as they contain nutrients, proteins, enzymes, and growth factors naturally found in the adrenal glands that are needed for regeneration and repair. It provides the building blocks for the body's own adrenal glands to support optimal function.

Adrenal glandular products are extracted from the adrenal tissues of free range, grass-fed cows usually from New Zealand and supply both the adrenal medulla and cortex.

It is best to work with a qualified practitioner before supplementing with adrenal glandular products to ensure they are suitable for you personally.

Just stop and breathe

When you are on the infertility rollercoaster of emotion or with any form of stress or overwhelm, it is important to take time out each day to just sit in silence and breathe.

So, stop now, if you can. Close your eyes and take a slow deep breath in for the count of four. Hold your breath for the count of four and then exhale slowly to the count of seven before you open your eyes. You should feel much calmer and relaxed. I find this breathing technique provides instant stress relief when life gets crazy.

Aim to pause and breathe at least two or three times a day. You don't have to do it for long as just a few minutes will be enough to calm your nervous system.

Meditation and fertility

One of the biggest lessons of my 10-year fertility journey is that I wish I had started meditation earlier. In fact, it was only about five years ago that meditation became a regular part of my routine after a friend recommended to me the *Headspace* app. I committed to 10 minutes a day and, to be honest, initially I found it really difficult. During the meditation, I had so many thoughts going around in my head that I wondered if I was doing it right, as I just couldn't switch off. Despite this, I kept persevering, and after two weeks of committing to 10 minutes a day, I found myself able to transition into a calm, happy, safe place every time I meditated. I then extended my practice and focused on positive visualisation, which again I found hard at first, but it became easier with practice.

Meditation is so important for anyone who is suffering from infertility, as often, we are in a dark place reluctant to open up and communicate with friends and family around us. I frequently experienced overwhelming disappointment month after month, along with frustration towards myself, fear of failure, and envy towards those who seemed to be able to conceive effortlessly. Meditation helped me focus on the positives instead of negative self-talk, and I became more able to pick up on the subtle signs the universe was trying to tell me.

Practicing meditation helped me to take a step back and see how my negative thoughts and feelings were affecting my physical body. We must recognize the connection between our mind and body and take care of our emotional health in order for our bodies to work efficiently. This is especially true with reproductive health, as if we are in a state of stress, our hormones go out of balance and our reproductive system literally shuts down. This is because getting pregnant is not considered essential for survival when we are in a fight-or-flight stress situation.

When we are less stressed, our hormones are more in harmony and we sleep better, which increases our chances of conceiving and maintaining a healthy pregnancy.

As I mentioned in chapter 5, the *Headspace* meditation app is one of the most popular apps on the market and is what I used. I think it is great. There are, however, plenty of other free fertility meditation apps on the market such as *Circle and Bloom* and *Expectful,* so have a search on the web for the latest apps and see what is best for you.

10 minutes a day is all you need to see positive changes in your stress levels and mindset, so why not give it a try?

Anxiety

It is quite common to suffer from anxiety when you are trying to conceive. If you find it gets worse in the second half of your cycle, then it could be because of a combination of high cortisol (because of stress) and low levels of the hormone progesterone, so it is important to get your hormones tested. This is because progesterone is known as our anti-anxiety hormone, as it has a calming and soothing effect on our emotions.

I used to get terrible anxiety around the time my period was due, especially if I suspected I might be pregnant. I remember being so terrified of going to the bathroom in case my period had turned up that I kept putting it off. When I finally got around to going to the bathroom, I would physically shake like I was having a panic attack. I know now that a combination of high cortisol and low progesterone was likely influencing this. Thyroid dysfunction can also cause anxiety, so it is important to get your thyroid tested if you are trying to conceive. I will go into more detail about thyroid dysfunction in the next chapter.

Do you have space for a baby?

During my fertility journey, I believed that my future baby was waiting for the right moment, for me to be ready when everything was aligned, and the timing was right. This was one belief that kept me going all those years despite the negative test results and early pregnancy losses.

Consider these questions: do you have space for a baby? Could a baby easily slot into your lifestyle at the moment? Do you have the physical or emotional energy to get pregnant or raise a baby? Are you in a suitable position financially? If you answer no to any of these questions, then it is time for some self-reflection. Is there anything you can let go of to free up more time? What can you do to support your physical and emotional energy?

For me, I created space by giving up my permanent job, which was a job that was quite draining and not very fulfilling. I quit my job to build my nutrition clinic. Having this new sense of purpose and extra time on my hands helped to reduce my stress levels and anxiety and I feel this was one of the pivotal reasons I could conceive at age 43, although not the only one. What can you do to create space for a baby in your life?

Infertility burnout

The World Health Organisation (WHO) defines burnout as an "occupational phenomenon" a state of physical and emotional exhaustion resulting from long-term stress. In today's world, burnout is a common topic of discussion, especially when it comes to demanding careers like doctors, CEOs, lawyers, nurses, caregivers, and individuals who have a full daily schedule of one-to-one clients.

Burnout can also be a factor for couples who have experienced long-term infertility challenges and failed IVF procedures. Any practitioner taking on a new client who has been trying to conceive for more than 12 months should assess them for infertility burnout.

What is infertility burnout?

Infertility burnout occurs when you experience mental, physical, and emotional exhaustion because of the stress of trying to get pregnant. As a result, you may feel overwhelmed and unable to cope. Infertility burnout is something to be aware of if you have been experiencing infertility and recurrent miscarriage for a long time.

We are designed to cope with the little stressors of our daily lives and when they resolve, we go back to a state of homeostasis, which is a natural state of balance. 'Homeostasis is defined as a self-regulating process by which a living organism can maintain internal stability while adjusting to changing internal conditions. Homeostasis is not static or unvarying, it is a dynamic process that can change internal conditions as required to survive external challenges.'[3]

We can only deal with these constant stressors for so long and when we reach our limit, this is when burnout tends to occur.

With infertility, the stressors are constant. Each cycle that you are trying to conceive you start off the two weeks before ovulation with a sense of hope and optimism and if you don't conceive that cycle, you then feel crushed and disappointed. Now imagine experiencing that month after month for years. It was 10 years in my case.

As well as the monthly stressors of managing your cycle, making sure you don't miss your fertility window, dealing with the impatience of the two weeks wait, and the stress of taking a pregnancy test, there are also for many couples a few major stressors thrown in as well. These are stressors such as IVF procedures and injections, miscarriages, D and C procedures, frequent blood tests and appointments, all of which take their toll after a while.

The problem is that when we reach the stage of burnout, it will have serious implications for our fertility, especially our hormones, as discussed earlier in this chapter. Burnout makes it a very challenging internal environment for conception, so it becomes a vicious cycle.

After 10 years of trying to conceive my second child, I felt that after a while, my body developed a coping mechanism that blocked my emotions whenever I suffered an early pregnancy loss. After several years of experiencing multiple chemical pregnancies, I felt numb each time one occurred. I just thought "oh well, that was that then" and just got on with it. I always poured myself a glass of wine and tucked into some food that I had been avoiding as comfort, but I couldn't cry. I just felt numb. When you reach the point of infertility burnout, here is how you might feel:

- Exhausted on all levels, mentally, emotionally, physically

- That you want to hide away and be alone, not wanting to see or talk to people

- A lack of motivation and interest in daily activities

- Anger and jealousy at others, especially if there are new baby announcements

- Wanting to sleep but struggling to

- Anxiety, sadness, and depression

- Feeling overwhelmed and unable to cope

- Blaming self and seeing self as a failure

- Pretending to be fine to others when you are not.

Steps to help yourself

- If you are offered a fertility counsellor through your fertility clinic, take it up. Talking things out with a professional can really help and good counsellors are hard to find.

- Take a month off trying to conceive and plan a schedule of fun non fertility related activities you enjoy. For example, going to the movies, walking in nature, getting a facial or massage to pamper yourself, read a good book, go to exercise classes, take up a creative hobby, go out for drinks or dinner with friends. Anything non fertility related that is going to make you smile.

- My list of non-fertility related activities included: Les Mills classes at the gym, yoga, meditation, making new recipes, going for walks, reading my Outlander book collection and studying nutrition. During the first few years of my fertility journey, I was studying nutritional science, which occupied my mind, so I didn't constantly think about getting pregnant.

- If you have been trying to conceive for a while and you are starting to show signs of burnout, think about taking an extended break of around three months to reset. I know it is hard to do, especially when you are over 40 and you don't want to waste any time, but it might be exactly what you need. It is a chance to refresh, reset, heal, and deal with any imbalances or health issues. After a break, you can resume trying to conceive with a renewed sense of energy and optimism.

- Find a support group of like-minded people going through the same thing as you, not your friends or family, as they won't truly understand what you are going through. Look for online fertility forums and Facebook groups.

- Take a digital detox. If you have just received bad news, take at least a week off social media. Comparisonitis can be a common feeling when you are experiencing infertility. The constant bombardment of pregnancy and baby announcements and cute photos on social media makes it difficult to stay positive. Taking a week or more off all social media platforms protects you from all the negative news you don't want to hear. Without the distractions on social media, you develop the strength to continue.

- Consider introducing the stress management tools I discussed earlier in this chapter, such as deep breathing, yoga, meditation and bathing in Epsom salts.

Chapter summary

Here are some actions you can take to implement the key points of this chapter:

- Ensure you are supporting your adrenal glands daily with nutrients that are needed for the synthesis of adrenal hormones but also nutrients that will regulate cortisol levels. Key nutrients like vitamin C, vitamin B5, and magnesium are necessary to support your adrenals daily and are depleted more rapidly during periods of stress.

- Taking supplements is not enough to address stress levels when you are on the infertility rollercoaster. Taking the time each day for activities you enjoy as well as stress management tools such as restorative yoga, meditation and going for walks in nature are all important ways to balance your stress levels.

- If you are suffering from infertility burnout, consider taking a break from trying to conceive for a month or two as a chance to reset. If needed, seek the support from a counsellor who works with infertility patients. Your fertility clinic or organisations like Fertility New Zealand (if you live in New Zealand) can put you in touch with recommended counsellors.

Chapter Eight

Could it be your thyroid?

An underactive thyroid, or hypothyroidism, is very common in females and can be an undetected cause of infertility and recurrent pregnancy loss. Hyperthyroidism (an overactive thyroid) can also be problematic but is not as common, so I am going to focus mainly on hypothyroidism in this chapter. However, I will close off this chapter with some key information on hyperthyroidism and what you can do if you have this condition and are trying to get pregnant.

I spent 10 years trying to get pregnant with baby number two and during this time, I often had a gut feeling that I was having issues with my thyroid. Despite my gut feeling, it was hard to prove as the limited tests that my doctor and fertility specialist were prepared to do at the time (just TSH and T4) always came back within the normal range. This is a worldwide problem that affects many women, as conventional thyroid testing unfortunately cannot give a full picture of what is going on with the thyroid. Consequently, many women live their lives with undetected subclinical hypothyroidism, wondering why they are experiencing symptoms such as fatigue, hair loss, constipation and weight gain.

What may be causing your thyroid dysfunction?

Thyroid issues are one of the biggest challenges with unexplained infertility, as they often go undiagnosed. There may be a chance that you have a thyroid dysfunction even though your doctor has tested your thyroid and says it is normal. Most doctors just test your thyroid-stimulating hormone (TSH) which is a hormone produced by the pituitary gland that instructs your thyroid to make thyroid hormone. This is only part of the picture though and doesn't show whether the active thyroid hormone is actually getting into your cells and doing what is it meant to do.

There are several ways your thyroid may be affected so it is beneficial to work with a qualified practitioner to help to identify the root cause. Some of the most common causes of thyroid dysfunction are:

Stress

As mentioned in the previous chapter, when we are suffering from long-term stress, which is common with infertility, our thyroid is down regulated as it is not considered an essential function during the high alert stress state. Because of this, our body slows down our metabolism to conserve energy. We know this as subclinical hypothyroidism or functional hypothyroidism and it reflects a dysfunction or miscommunication in the hypothalamus, pituitary and adrenal (HPA) axis, as opposed to a problem with the thyroid itself. The important thing here is to support the whole glandular system rather than just supporting the thyroid gland in isolation. Treating the thyroid without supporting the adrenal glands may make symptoms worse.

This was a huge issue for me, and it is likely the main reason I had thyroid issues. As a chronic asthmatic and person living with eczema, I spent over 20 years using various steroid medications on and off. Long-term steroid use depletes adrenal function, so I had to work hard to keep my adrenals in a healthy balance. Allergies are also stressful for the body, although we rarely think of health conditions as actual stressors, but they are. Our bodies are constantly working hard to maintain homeostasis whilst being under threat from allergens.

Nutritional deficiencies

The second reason for thyroid dysfunction is vitamin and mineral deficiencies, as they can affect the production of thyroid hormone, especially if you are deficient in iodine and the amino acid tyrosine. Nutritional deficiencies can also affect the conversion of the inactive thyroid hormone T4 (thyroxine) to the active thyroid hormone T3 (triiodothyronine) in the liver. The important nutrients that support this conversion in the liver are zinc, selenium, iron, and vitamin D. I will cover this in more detail later in this chapter.

Autoimmunity

The third reason, and this is the most common cause, is that your thyroid dysfunction may be caused by autoimmunity, yet you are unlikely to know this if your doctor only tests your TSH. The only way of knowing whether your thyroid is under attack from your overactive immune system is by testing thyroid antibodies, yet most doctors will not test for this. This is a worldwide problem. Testing thyroid antibodies alerts us to whether there is an autoimmune attack on your thyroid, and this may manifest as either Hashimoto's thyroiditis (underactive) and Graves' disease (overactive). For some people, and I am one of them, it is not so clear cut as you can swing from being both underactive and overactive at different times, which makes it so hard to diagnose. This is a pattern typical of autoimmune thyroid disease and the root cause is essentially the same for both (gut health plays a huge part) so treating the root cause of the autoimmunity is the treatment priority.

A stressful event can sometimes trigger autoimmunity, such as a major illness, stress, trauma, infection, or pregnancy. This occurs against a background of genetic predisposition, (as autoimmunity has a tendency to run in families) along with gut health and immune function.

Poor gut health

There are several factors that can create an internal environment that promotes inflammation and autoimmunity. These can be:

- Intestinal permeability (otherwise known as leaky gut)

- Chronic infections such as candida (a common yeast overgrowth), bacterial vaginosis or small intestinal bacterial overgrowth (SIBO). These may need to be treated with specific antimicrobials.

- Food sensitivities.

As discussed in chapter 4, researchers have found a connection between gluten intolerance and the autoimmune thyroid conditions Hashimoto's and Graves' disease. This is because thyroid tissue is very similar to gluten in terms of its molecular structure, so the overactive immune system gets confused and attacks thyroid tissue, mistaking it for gluten.

With autoimmune thyroid conditions, the standard blood tests of TSH and T4 are often within the normal range. Therefore, you are told by your doctor that your thyroid is normal, even when you still have symptoms of thyroid dysfunction. Testing for thyroid antibodies is the only way to uncover autoimmune thyroid as the number of antibodies reflects the severity of the immune attack on your thyroid. Unfortunately, doctors seldom conduct tests for thyroid antibodies, causing many women to believe that their thyroid is normal, even though they are still experiencing symptoms of low thyroid function. I see this in my clinic all the time, my clients just cannot understand why they are losing hair and putting on weight. When I mention the thyroid, they always respond with "My doctor tested my thyroid and said it was normal." However, when I see a copy of the results, most times the doctor has only tested TSH.

Postpartum depletion and postpartum thyroiditis

Pregnancy can also trigger postpartum thyroid problems. It is common for women to develop a thyroid condition in the months after giving birth, called postpartum thyroiditis. This can occur when the stress of a pregnancy and the postpartum period overwhelms the immune system of the mother and causes inflammation of the thyroid gland. Although this typically occurs within the first year of giving birth, it can occur many years later.

Although I was never tested at the time, I believe I was suffering from postpartum thyroiditis after the birth of my son, who is now 15. In hindsight, it makes sense, as I had most of the symptoms such as low body temperature, weight gain, fatigue, and the inability to lose weight after pregnancy and breastfeeding despite a healthy diet and regular exercise programme.

I covered postpartum thyroiditis in detail in chapter 2, as it is a common cause of secondary infertility. Screening for postpartum thyroiditis should be a routine part of preconception screening if you are trying for another child, but it is not.

During the preconception period, it's vital to have a full thyroid panel completed, since the thyroid has to work twice as hard during pregnancy. If we do not support the thyroid going into pregnancy with nutrient building blocks, a diet that reduces autoimmune triggers, healthy gut function, reduced stress levels and, if necessary, thyroid medication, then problems may occur. The thyroid may struggle to keep up with the extra demands of pregnancy and this may sadly result in complications such as miscarriage for some people.

If you have a thyroid condition and you are concerned about your thyroid in the early stages of pregnancy, ask your doctor to test your thyroid function regularly during the first trimester and if your numbers start to look a bit concerning then your doctor can intervene with treatment.

Tests via your doctor

When your doctor completes a blood test to check your thyroid function, they will mostly only test TSH (thyroid-stimulating hormone) and if there is an abnormality with TSH, then they will test free T4 (the thyroid hormone thyroxine).

TSH is a pituitary hormone that stimulates the thyroid gland to produce thyroid hormone when needed. TSH ideally needs to be between 1.0 and 2.0 mIU/L for optimal function, anything above 2.5 mIU/L indicates some level of hypothyroidism. The problem is many women have normal TSH levels and still have symptoms of low thyroid function. Unfortunately, in these cases testing just TSH highlights what the pituitary gland is doing, and not the actual function of the thyroid. Testing just free T4 (thyroxine) as well isn't really a reliable indicator of thyroid function as T4 is an inactive hormone that needs to be converted to T3 (triiodothyronine) to become active. So, testing free T3, the active thyroid hormone is going to give a better picture of your thyroid function.

Unfortunately, it is often challenging to get a free T3 test from your doctor, unless you push really hard for a full thyroid panel, and it is not always easy. This is why so many women have undiagnosed subclinical thyroid problems.

Luckily, nowadays, you can request a free T3 test as part of a full comprehensive thyroid panel in many countries through a naturopath, nutritionist, or functional medicine practitioner.

Several factors can impair the conversion of T4 to T3 in the liver. These are aging, inflammation, stress, severe injury, calorie restriction, fasting, poor gut health, an imbalance of gut bacteria, chemical or toxic metal exposure, a lack of antioxidants, increased free radical damage, nutrient deficiency, high alcohol intake, liver or kidney disease, severe illness, and surgery. If you have concerns that you may have any of these issues, I recommend you work with a nutritionist, naturopath or functional medicine practitioner.

I pushed for full thyroid testing frequently, and my doctor said she would run the tests. When I asked for the results on these occasions, it frustrated me to discover that they had only tested the TSH and free T4. You really need to be your own advocate and push really hard to get the tests done and ask for a copy of your results. Please don't just accept over the phone that they are in the normal range.

The full comprehensive thyroid panel test also includes thyroid antibodies, which are important to test for Hashimoto's thyroiditis or Grave's disease. The two main antibodies tested are anti-microsomal antibody Ab or thyroid peroxidase (TPOAb) and anti-thyroglobulin antibody (TgAb). Hashimoto's and Grave's disease are autoimmune conditions in females that can contribute to fertility problems, although Hashimoto's is the most common. Testing for thyroid antibodies is also important to do if there is a family history of other autoimmune conditions, such as coeliac disease. In both Hashimoto's thyroiditis and Grave's disease, the thyroid blood tests may show normal results in the early stages of the disease, but elevated antibodies suggest an immune attack on the thyroid gland. If left untreated, the thyroid blood tests may gradually become abnormal over time.

Reverse T3

A comprehensive thyroid panel will also test for reverse T3 (RT3), which is an inactive form of T3. In a normal healthy person, the body converts T4 into both T3 and RT3 and can quickly eliminate RT3. In some situations, the production of RT3 increases as a protective mechanism, which reduces levels of the active T3 in the body. This slows down metabolism and causes hypothyroid symptoms, which is also known as thyroid resistance.

The key issue with high levels of RT3 is that it will bind to T3 receptor sites in the body, but because it is inactive, it has no activity. So essentially, high RT3 levels can give you symptoms of hypothyroidism, even though your TSH and free T4 are within the normal range.

What causes high levels of reverse T3?

The main causes of high RT3 levels are:

- Stress as cortisol increases the conversion of T4 into RT3

- Chronic infections and inflammation

- Low-calorie diets.

If you have a high RT3 blood test result, then your focus needs to be on reducing your stress levels in any way you can and making sure you are eating well, not on a restricted low-calorie or too low-carb diet. Remember stress is not just being busy. If you have an infection, gut issue, or food intolerance that is causing inflammation and uncomfortable symptoms, this is stressful for your body as well.

Checking your basal body temperature

A simple test you can do at home to check your thyroid function is to take your basal body temperature with a thermometer upon waking for five days in a row. This is best done between day 5 and 14 of the menstrual cycle. A normal basal body temperature falls within the range of 36.4 to 37.0 degrees Celsius. If it is consistently below 36.0 in the 35.5–35.9 range, then that could mean that you have an underactive thyroid, as a lower body temperature indicates a slow metabolism.

What are the common symptoms of low thyroid function?

The symptoms of hypothyroidism can be similar to those of various other conditions, but the most common symptoms include:

- Fatigue and exhaustion

- Unexplained weight gain

- Hair loss, outer third of eyebrow missing

- Dry skin, brittle nails

- Poor concentration

- Enlarged thyroid gland (goitre)

- Inability to lose weight

- Cold hands and feet, chills, feels the cold

- Constipation.

Supporting the thyroid with key nutrients

Nutritional deficiencies can be a cause of an underactive thyroid as nutrients such as iodine, tyrosine, selenium, zinc, iron, and vitamin D are essential for the function of the thyroid. To support the manufacture of thyroid hormones and the conversion of inactive thyroid hormone T4 to the active T3 hormone, we need the following nutrients daily:

Iodine

The trace mineral iodine is essential for the production of thyroid hormones, along with the amino acid tyrosine. It is recommended to supplement with at least 150 mcg a day as potassium iodide. Good food sources are seafood, seaweed such as kelp and bladderwrack, kombu, nori, Celtic Sea salt or iodised salt.

Tyrosine

The amino acid tyrosine is also essential for manufacturing thyroid hormones, along with the trace mineral iodine. Eating protein with each meal is your best source, although supplementing with tyrosine as part of a thyroid support supplement may help to support thyroid function. In most thyroid supplements, the dose is around 250–500 mg a day. Good food sources are dairy foods, poultry, fish, red meat, eggs, almonds, avocados, and bananas.

Selenium

The trace mineral selenium is an essential component of the enzyme that converts T4 to T3 in the liver. 150 mcg a day is the recommended dose, and it is important not to exceed a maximum of 200 mcg a day from all sources. Under the care of a qualified practitioner, higher doses may be prescribed as part of an autoimmune protocol. Good food sources are Brazil nuts, salmon, chicken, brown rice, beef, and walnuts.

Zinc

The mineral zinc is involved in thyroid hormone production and the conversion of the inactive thyroid hormone T4 to the active thyroid hormone T3 in the liver. If you have low zinc and are supplementing, 30 mg a day is a beneficial dose. Good food sources are oysters, beef, chicken, dairy, cashews, almonds and pumpkin seeds.

Iron

Iron is another mineral that is very important for healthy thyroid function as it is involved in the production of TSH and the conversion of T4 to T3. If you have low iron and are supplementing, 24 mg a day is the recommended daily dose. Good food sources are beef, lamb, pork, and liver. Animal sources contain haem iron, which has higher absorption. Beetroot, spinach, kale, beans, lentils, tofu, molasses, and dried fruit are all non-haem plant-based sources with lower absorption.

Eating foods rich in vitamin C with iron food sources can help improve absorption. Citrus fruits, strawberries, broccoli, capsicum, and potatoes are all rich sources.

Vitamin D

Studies have shown that patients with Hashimoto's thyroiditis, the autoimmune thyroid condition, have lower vitamin D levels than the general population. In a Greek study, Hashimoto's thyroiditis patients who were deficient in vitamin D took 1,200–4,000 iu of vitamin D every day for four months after which they had significantly lower levels of anti-thyroid antibodies. [1]

It is therefore beneficial to consider vitamin D as a supplement if you have an autoimmune thyroid condition, and for fertility in general, as vitamin D is important for your whole glandular system and approximately one fifth of the global population is deficient in vitamin D. Taking around 2,000 iu daily is a general recommendation for thyroid support and fertility, but testing is a good idea as you may need more than this.

Additional support

It is staggering how many women are suffering from symptoms of low thyroid function despite being told that their blood tests are normal. If you suspect you have a thyroid problem, it is worth ensuring you are getting adequate levels of these nutrients daily, which will help your thyroid manufacture and convert hormones.

It is also important to avoid compounds that can block the absorption of iodine by binding to iodine receptors in the thyroid gland. These are:

- Raw brassicas in excess because they contain a compound called goitrogens, which can block iodine absorption. Cooking or fermenting is fine.

- Unfiltered water, because of fluoride and chloride, which are chemicals that can bind to iodine receptors and impair iodine absorption.

Initially, researchers believed that soy consumption negatively affected thyroid function by increasing TSH levels, but more recent studies have changed this advice. 'A 2022 review of 417 studies found soy isoflavones do not have a negative effect on thyroid function, thyroid hormone levels or reproductive hormones.' [2]

In terms of dietary recommendations, consider adopting a gluten-free diet if you are experiencing unexplained infertility and you suspect you may have a thyroid problem. Many studies have linked gluten consumption to both Hashimoto's thyroiditis and Grave's disease, the autoimmune thyroid conditions.

You can download my free guide on *Getting Started with Gluten Free* from www.nutritionforhealthnz.com/home.

Just a final note of caution. It is important not to supplement with high doses of iodine to support your thyroid function unless you are under the care of a qualified practitioner. High doses may cause your underactive thyroid to tip over into an overactive hyperthyroid state, which can be harmful. I learned this the hard way when I was a nutrition student, and I experimented with different supplements as you do. At one point, I felt like I was swinging between a hypo and hyperthyroid state. If you develop anxiety, have problems sleeping, or develop heart palpitations, this could be a sign you are taking too much iodine.

Hyperthyroidism

Hyperthyroidism is another thyroid condition that can affect fertility. Although not as common as hypothyroidism, it is still worth a mention as I close this chapter on thyroid conditions.

What is hyperthyroidism?

Hyperthyroidism is a condition where the thyroid becomes overactive and produces too much thyroid hormone. Whilst most females suffering from infertility have issues with hypothyroidism, we still need to consider hyperthyroidism, as having an overactive thyroid can also lead to infertility issues. It approximately affects around 2% of women.

The main issue with hyperthyroidism is that it can lead to malnutrition and excessive weight loss. This is because thyroid hormone levels are consistently too high, which speeds up metabolism and all body processes. As a result, the body ends up burning through and depleting nutrients quickly.

The most common cause of hyperthyroidism is the autoimmune condition Grave's disease, which your doctor would diagnose with a blood test to identify elevated autoantibodies. Patients with hyperthyroidism usually have low levels of thyroid-stimulating hormone (TSH), usually less than 0.30 ml/UL and elevated levels of T4 and T3.

According to functional medicine doctor Amy Myers, in her book *The Autoimmune Solution,* In Graves' disease, an antibody known as thyrotropin receptor antibody (TRAb) can mimic pituitary hormones and completely override the system, causing an overactive thyroid. [3]

With Graves' disease, you may also develop thyroid peroxidase (TPO) or anti-thyroglobulin antibodies. Some of the common symptoms of hyperthyroidism include:

- Heart palpitations and a fast heart rate

- Increased sweating and feeling sensitive to the heat

- Increased appetite

- Weight loss

- Trouble falling asleep

- Anxiety, nervousness, and panic attacks

- Loose, frequent bowel motions

- Fatigue and weakness, including muscle weakness and tremors

- Goitre (although this is not always present)

- Bulging eyes

- Lighter menstrual periods

- Shortness of breath.

As with hypothyroidism, there are several underlying factors which can lead to the development of hyperthyroidism. These are:

Gluten and molecular mimicry

With all autoimmune diseases, there appears to be a connection with gluten, because of a process called molecular mimicry. This is when the proteins of gluten share a very similar molecule structure with the proteins of your thyroid gland. So, when you eat gluten regularly, the immune system gets confused and starts attacking the tissues of your thyroid gland. This is because the protein building blocks are very similar.

Iodine intake

Carefully monitoring iodine intake is important, as insufficient amounts can lead to goitre and hypothyroidism, while excessive amounts can cause hyperthyroidism. An iodine patch test using Lugol's iodine solution can be a useful way of ensuring iodine intake is optimal and not excessive.

How to do an iodine patch test

Using Lugol's iodine, paint a coin size patch on your skin after your shower once a day. If it absorbs completely, paint another patch on your skin the next day. Watch how long it takes to fade and disappear completely, which is a sign it is being absorbed by the skin. Continue daily until it no longer absorbs and is still visible after 24 hours. This is a sign that your iodine is optimal as the body uptakes only what it needs from the skin. In New Zealand, individuals can only purchase Lugol's iodine through a qualified practitioner because of regulations.

Gut health

As intestinal permeability is often the root cause of most autoimmune conditions, working to nourish and heal the gut lining and eliminate underlying infections is important. Revisit chapter four for more information on gut health.

Here are some nutrients that may help to support an overactive thyroid:

L-carnitine

There have been studies that suggest that l-carnitine may help to reduce hyperthyroid symptoms such as insomnia, nervousness, heart palpitations, and tremors. This is because l-carnitine inhibits the entry of both triiodothyronine (T3) and thyroxine (T4) into the cell nuclei [4]

Red meat, dairy products, fish, and poultry are the best dietary sources of l-carnitine; however, additional supplementation may be required to reduce more severe hyperthyroid symptoms. It is best to work with a qualified practitioner on dosing rather than experimenting yourself.

Coenzyme Q10

Studies have linked hyperthyroidism with reduced circulating levels of coenzyme Q10 and that hyperthyroid patients have the lowest levels of coenzyme Q10 of all human diseases.

This highlights the benefit of coenzyme Q10 for all aspects of fertility. As well as being a potent antioxidant, increasing fertility, supporting mitochondrial health and improving egg quality (as discussed in chapter 6), coenzyme Q10 as ubiquinol can also be helpful to take as a supplement if you have hyperthyroidism.

Lemon balm tea

Drinking lemon balm tea regularly can have a calming effect on the thyroid and can reduce feelings of anxiety and nervousness.

Chapter summary

Here are some actions you can take to implement the key points of this chapter:

- Ensure you are supporting your thyroid daily with the key nutrient building blocks that are needed for the synthesis of thyroid hormones and the conversion of the inactive thyroid hormone T4 to the active thyroid hormone T3 in the liver. These are iodine, tyrosine, zinc, selenium, iron, and vitamin D.

- Work with a functional medicine doctor, naturopath, or nutritionist to get a full comprehensive thyroid panel completed, which will give you an accurate picture of what is going on with your thyroid. Ensure that the comprehensive thyroid panel includes testing for TSH, free T4, free T3, reverse T3, and thyroid antibodies.

- If you have an autoimmune thyroid condition, then it is important to adopt a gluten-free diet. This is because many studies have linked gluten consumption to autoimmunity because of molecular mimicry, where the immune system confuses proteins of gluten with thyroid tissue. Also, consider working with a practitioner to investigate and eliminate additional food intolerances and heal the gut lining. If you are reacting to any foods, even healthy foods, then this could trigger the immune system to overreact, which could lead to inflammation and autoimmunity.

- Stress is also a factor that may be down regulating your thyroid gland. Support the hypothalamus, pituitary, adrenal axis (HPA) axis first, and not just the thyroid in isolation. Revisit chapter 7 on ways to support stress and adrenal function.

Chapter Nine

Silent low grade inflammation and immune dysregulation

I spent some time researching silent low-grade inflammation and its role in unexplained infertility and recurrent pregnancy loss, trying to understand the connection. In my research, I discovered that many women with unexplained infertility and recurrent pregnancy loss may have an immune system imbalance with a pattern of elevated Th17 immune cells and decreased T regulatory cells. This is an imbalance that often occurs with chronic inflammation and autoimmunity. The immune system is complex with many players, but this pattern is worth noting as this Th17/T regulatory cell imbalance can be influenced by our diet, lifestyle and environment. Also, the key player in all the complexities of our immune orchestra is the gut microbiome.

Unexplained infertility

Unexplained infertility is a term used when there is no obvious physiological reason that you cannot get pregnant, despite standard testing and scans from your doctor or fertility clinic. According to *Fertility New Zealand*, unexplained infertility affects approximately 15 – 25% of infertile couples.

I know firsthand how hopeless it feels to be told you have unexplained infertility. For 10 years, this was my journey with over 17 chemical pregnancies and three miscarriages at around six to eight weeks. Despite being told at age 41 (after my IVF ended in miscarriage) that my only hope was to use a donor egg, I conceived naturally at age 43. I had a healthy pregnancy and gave birth to my miracle baby girl at age 44.

When your doctor first tells you that you have unexplained infertility, it seems a relief that there is nothing actually wrong with you or your partner. Most doctors recommend IVF or other assisted reproductive treatment as the next steps when you have unexplained infertility. However, for many couples like myself, IVF doesn't fix the unexplained infertility issue and the heartache and frustration continues, but without a sense of direction and hope.

Is silent low-grade inflammation the cause

Silent low-grade inflammation may be barely noticeable to you with only mild, easy to ignore symptoms such as a skin rash, asthma, reflux or abdominal discomfort. Although the symptoms are manageable and not that troublesome, under the surface, your symptoms may be permanently triggering the adaptive immune system and creating inflammation. Long-term activation of the adaptive immune system can lead to autoimmunity and a lack of self-tolerance, which means the body cannot identify the difference between cells and tissues that are self and non-self, and so attacks itself. I will explain more about this later.

Researchers estimate that silent, low-grade inflammation can cause up to 50% of cases of unexplained infertility. If this is you, check in with yourself to see what symptoms you are experiencing and whether working to resolve your chronic condition can help to enhance your fertility.

Acute and chronic inflammation

Inflammation is an important, natural response of the body to protect itself against harm, which may come from an irritant, cut, injury, or pathogen. There are two types of inflammation: acute and chronic.

Acute inflammation

Acute inflammation is the rapid response of the body when a cut or injury occurs. White blood cells swarm to the area of the injury, cut or infection, causing redness, pain and swelling. The cells involved in this inflammatory response trap bacteria and help the healing process. Inflammation is an essential immune response to protect the area and prevent injuries and infections from getting worse and spreading. Once the injury or infection heals, the body usually resolves inflammation.

Chronic inflammation

If acute inflammation doesn't resolve itself quickly and remains untreated, it may lead to chronic inflammation as the immune system becomes continually activated. Long-term exposure to environmental toxins, irritants, infections and food sensitivities that trigger the immune system can also cause chronic inflammation. This may manifest in the body as:

- Pain anywhere in the body (joints, stomach, back, chest, etc.)

- Fatigue

- Skin rashes, eczema, psoriasis

- Asthma

- Endometriosis or PCOS

- IBS or inflammatory bowel disease

If we ignore chronic inflammation and let it persist, it can tip us over the threshold into autoimmunity, which is where tissue destruction starts to occur. This is when the immune system goes awry and attacks healthy body cells and tissues, essentially attacking itself. Examples of this are the autoimmune condition rheumatoid arthritis, where inflammatory cytokines attack the tissues of the joints or the tissues of the thyroid with Hashimoto's thyroiditis.

How can chronic inflammation affect fertility?

1. Chronic inflammation can damage reproductive cells and tissues such as the egg, uterus, ovaries and sperm.

2. Chronic inflammation can be the driver of an autoimmune response in the body in which elevated antibodies cause the body to attack its own tissues, which may include a fetus.

Inflammation and oxidative stress have a close relationship, and high levels of oxidative stress can cause unexplained infertility. Oxidative stress occurs when there is an imbalance of free radicals and antioxidants in the body. Free radicals are created by factors such as a poor diet, stress, smoking, alcohol and excessive exercise. An antioxidant rich diet helps to prevent free radical damage to cells and DNA, which is why a high intake of brightly coloured vegetables and fruit are an important part of a fertility diet.

Autoimmunity

Researchers estimate that up to half of women with unexplained infertility and/or recurrent pregnancy loss have issues with autoimmunity, but they may not even be aware of it. This occurs when there is an imbalance in the adaptive (acquired) immune system. The common patterns seen with autoimmunity are an imbalance in Th1/Th2 immune cells, elevated Th17 cells and a reduction of T regulatory cells (T regs), which help to calm down the overactive immune response.

T helper 1/T helper 2 ratio

The immune system has two major arms, T helper 1 and T helper 2 cells. Our gut microbiome plays an important role in keeping these two arms of the immune system in a healthy balance. A dominance of T helper 1 cells is associated with various autoimmune conditions and researchers have also linked T helper 2 dominance to more allergic conditions, such as asthma and hay fever.

For a successful pregnancy, the Th1/Th2 balance needs to shift towards Th2 dominance, a protective mechanism so that the immune system doesn't attack the baby.

'While in the pregnancy, Th1 cells inhibit the invasion of a trophoblastic cell, Th2 cells modulate a Th1 response, promote the trophoblast invasion and maintain the fetus.' [1] The trophoblast cells are the major cell type of the placenta that makes the hormone human chorionic gonadotropin (HCG) to ensure the endometrium will be receptive to the embryo during implantation. So, if the immune system is leaning too heavily towards Th1 dominance, there is a chance that implantation will fail.

Th17 cells

In cases of unexplained infertility and recurrent pregnancy loss, there is often an increase in Th17 cells. The function of Th17 cells is to facilitate the immune response against extracellular bacterial and fungal infections. Th17 cells promote inflammation, which not only creates an unreceptive environment for implantation, but plays a key role in the development of autoimmunity. 'Collectively, Th17 cells are highly potent inflammatory cells that initiate tissue inflammation and induce the infiltration of other inflammatory cells into the target organ.' [2]

Studies have also linked high numbers of Th17 cells to fetus rejection and recurrent pregnancy loss. 'The proportion of Th17 cells in the peripheral blood and decidua were significantly higher in unexplained recurrent spontaneous abortion (URSA) patients, compared to normal, early pregnant women.' [3]

Regulatory T cells (T regs)

It is a decrease in regulatory T cells, along with the increase in Th17 cells, that is thought to contribute to unexplained infertility, especially implantation failure and recurrent pregnancy loss. Regulatory T cells are an important regulator to counteract the inflammatory effects of the Th17 cells. A healthy balance between the immune effector cells (Th17) and immune regulatory cells (regulatory T cells) is important for fertility and pregnancy success. T regulatory cells help to calm down autoimmunity and the overactivity of the immune system. 'Regulatory T cells (Treg) contribute to immune homeostasis by maintaining unresponsiveness to self-antigens and suppressing exaggerated immune responses.' [4]

What causes this imbalance in the adaptive immune system?

There are many causes of this breakdown in immune tolerance as a result of high Th17 cells and low regulatory T cells. Some of the most common ones are:

- Chronic infections – viral, bacterial, fungal

- Stress/oxidative stress

- Poor gut health, Intestinal permeability (leaky gut)

- Imbalanced gut microbiome (gut dysbiosis)

- Food intolerances

- Diet high in refined sugar and processed foods

- Diet low in antioxidants

- Nutritional deficiencies

- Poor sleep

- Environmental factors, such as toxins, allergies and chemicals

- Lifestyle factors such as smoking and excessive alcohol

- Too little or too much exercise

The Th17/T regulatory cell imbalance is fairly new research. In fact, one study I was reading to do some background research for this article is from 2023, which shows how new this information is.

When I was experiencing recurrent chemical pregnancies and miscarriages, I hadn't made the connection at the time that it could have been a lack of self-tolerance at the implantation stage. It now makes sense that in the absence of T regulatory cells to calm things down, the immune system may attack the fetus. A healthy balance between Th17 cells and T regulatory cells is therefore crucial to achieve implantation and to maintain a pregnancy until term.

Looking back, I have now realised that prior to conceiving my miracle baby at age 43; I was actually inadvertently increasing my T regulatory cells and reducing my Th17 cells, which may have helped calm down my overactive immune system that was contributing to implantation failure. I believe I achieved this by:

- Spending a few months on the GAPS diet healing my gut, replenishing my gut microbiome, and removing food sensitivities that triggered my immune system.

- I had increased my vitamin D supplement intake, as it was June in New Zealand when I conceived, which is winter.

- I used reishi mushroom to support my immune system during the winter. I was really just trying to build a robust immune system for the winter months and not really thinking about getting pregnant. Now that I have reviewed what these supplements can do, I believe reishi may have played a part in regulating my dysfunctional immune system and building self-tolerance.

I will go into more details shortly about each of these supplements and how they influence T regulatory cells along with a microbiome supportive diet.

Looking at research, it is clear that supporting T regulatory cell production is important for women suffering from implantation failure and recurrent pregnancy loss.

Increasing T regulatory cells (T regs)

T regulatory cells play an important role in immune homeostasis and help to suppress and calm down an overactive immune system. This may help to reduce inflammation and autoimmunity. Diet, lifestyle and the health of the gut microbiome play a key role in this.

Gut microbiome

The gut microbiome communicates with the immune cells in the gut associated lymphoid tissue (GALT) and plays an important role in regulating the balance of Th17 and T regulatory cells and other immune cells. The status of the gut microbiome can affect the levels of inflammatory Th17 cells, which become elevated when there is gut dysbiosis.

Th17 secretes IL 17 the proinflammatory cytokine when it tries to clear the body of bacterial or fungal infections. So having any unresolved, low-grade infections such as Candida Albicans (the pathogenic yeast overgrowth), urinary tract bacterial infections, or small intestinal bacterial overgrowth (SIBO), can upregulate Th17 cells and promote silent, low-grade inflammation. It is called silent as you may not be aware of it, or it is mild enough that you can happily just carry on with it. If left unresolved, this silent inflammation may lead to autoimmunity and a loss of self-tolerance, which is especially harmful for fertility. Self-tolerance is the ability of the immune system to recognise *self* (cells and self-producing antigens) as a non-threat and to identify and mount an appropriate response to *non-self*, foreign antigens. When the body loses its self-tolerance, it attacks itself, unable to differentiate between self and non-self.

When Th17 cells remain constantly elevated, it results in a shortage of T regulatory cells responsible for calming down and resolving the inflammatory immune response. T regulatory cells maintain immune tolerance by distinguishing self-antigens from foreign antigens.

Optimising our gut microbiome with prebiotic foods, probiotic foods and probiotic supplements are important for promoting a diverse gut microbiome, and for increasing T regulatory cells to dampen down an overactive immune system.

My approach was to increase microbiome diversity by rotating probiotics and fermented foods rather than taking the same isolated strains. My rotation included spore forming probiotics, multi-strain probiotics, and saccharomyces boullardi, a probiotic yeast. Rotating strains introduced diversity to my gut microbiome, and this worked well for me.

Spore forming probiotics were my favourite though as my gut felt healthier when I took these. Spore forming probiotics reconditions the gut by increasing microbial diversity and encouraging the growth of beneficial gut bacteria. They also help to reduce systemic inflammation by increasing butyrate production (more on butyrate later) and support immune modulation. Typical spore forming probiotic strains include bacillus coagulans (SC-208), bacillus indicus (HU36), bacillus licheniformis (SL-307), bacillus subtillus (HU58) and bacillus clausii (SC-109).

Diet

Diet has the biggest influence over the development of T regulatory cells. As food entering the digestive system is the largest source of foreign material to enter the body, it makes sense that what we eat will affect our immune system. What we eat also influences the composition of our gut microbiome. The foods that typically increase Th17 cells and promote inflammation are:

- Refined sugar and processed foods

- Excess trans fats

- Food intolerances such as gluten and dairy

The development of T regulatory cells depends highly on your nutritional status. Food intolerances that trigger an inflammatory immune response can also promote Th17 dominance and reduce T regulatory cells. Foods that increase T regulatory cells and calm down inflammation are:

Probiotic foods

Having a serving a day of a probiotic food such as sauerkraut, kimchi, kefir, probiotic yoghurt, kombucha and sourdough bread all help to nourish the gut and increase microbiome diversity.

Fibre

Dietary fibre can promote T regulatory cell development through the production of short-chain fatty acids (SCFAs). Fermentation of dietary fibre and resistant starches by our gut microbiome in the colon produces these short-chain fatty acids (SCFAs). 'The three predominant SCFAs, acetate, butyrate and propionate, ameliorate inflammatory diseases by regulating T reg function and frequency.' [5]

Eating a diet rich in fresh fruit and vegetables is one of the easiest ways to increase dietary fibre.

Butyrate

Butyrate is a short-chain fatty acid that plays an important role in modulating the gut microbiome, which has a regulatory effect on the immune system. 'Butyrate is the primary fuel source for the colonocyte where nearly 90% of generated butyrate is metabolised locally in the colon.' [6]

Butyrate is beneficial because it:

- Supports the integrity of the intestinal lining

- Modulates and inhibits pro-inflammatory cytokines, reducing inflammation

- Activates T regulatory cell production, which calms down an overactive immune system

- Assists with the production of anti-inflammatory cytokines such as IL 10

- Modulates the gut microbiome and its effect on the immune system

'Butyrate supports the integrity of the intestinal epithelial barrier by regulating the expression of tight junctional proteins and supporting intestinal mucus production.' [7]

A diet high in fermentable fibre boosts butyrate production because it fuels the short-chain fatty acid (SCFA) producing bacteria in the colon, allowing them to thrive. Vegetables, fruits, legumes, whole grains, rice, boiled potatoes (resistance starch) and prebiotic foods such as onions, garlic, asparagus and artichoke all fuel butyrate production.

Polyphenols

Foods rich in polyphenols such as red wine, dark chocolate, tea, coffee, and many coloured fruits and vegetables contain antioxidants that have prebiotic properties and exert anti-microbial action against pathogenic gut microbes.

Regular consumption of dietary polyphenols feeds our beneficial gut microbes and increases our microbiome diversity. The richer and more diverse your community of gut microbes is, the lower your risk of disease and allergies.

I am not suggesting you go mad with wine, coffee, and chocolate, but it is good to know there are some benefits to our gut microbiome for moderate consumption. Consuming berries, grapes, plums, oranges, kiwifruit, pomegranate, coffee, green tea, black tea, red wine, hazelnuts, almonds, walnuts, spinach, broccoli, red onion, asparagus, and carrots can provide beneficial prebiotic action because of their rich polyphenol content.

Cod liver oil

Researchers have found that both vitamin D and vitamin A increase T regulatory cells, and omega-3 is one of nature's greatest anti-inflammatories. A daily serving of cod liver oil packs a power punch of immune regulating and anti-inflammatory action as it is not only rich in omega-3 but also contains naturally occurring vitamin A and D.

Green tea

Not technically a food, but green tea has been shown in studies to increase T regulatory cell frequency. The polyphenol EGCG 'One of the beneficial compounds in green tea has the powerful ability to increase the number of regulatory T cells that play a key role in immune function and the suppression of autoimmune disease.' [8] It may therefore be beneficial to change your regular coffee or black tea to green tea.

Supplements that may help to support T regulatory cells

There are many things we can do naturally to support to production of T regulatory cells. In addition to the dietary suggestions, you may benefit from using the following supplements during the preconception and implantation stage to regulate your immune system and increase self-tolerance by increasing T regulatory cells.

Vitamin D

According to studies, supplementing with vitamin D may reduce inflammation and increase T regulatory cell function in both healthy individuals and patients with autoimmune disorders. In five trials of autoimmune disorders which measured the proportion of T regs, a higher proportion was observed in the vitamin D group compared to controls at 12 months in all but one trial.' [9]

As mentioned in chapter 3, the skin produces vitamin D3 (cholecalciferol) when exposed to the sun, however a lack of daily sun exposure, especially over the winter months, leads to lower vitamin D levels. Foods such as eggs, cod liver oil, mushrooms, fatty fish such as tuna and salmon, and cow's milk also contain vitamin D3, but it can be difficult to get enough through the diet.

A deficiency in vitamin D3 has been associated with various autoimmune conditions, as it has a modulating effect on the immune system. As many fertility issues can result from an underlying autoimmune condition, it is important to get your vitamin D levels checked.

The general recommendation is to spend 15 minutes every day out in the sunshine with no sunscreen in the summer and at least an hour during the winter to allow your skin the opportunity to make vitamin D. In summer, it is best to avoid the heat of the day, so before 10.00 am and after 3.00 pm is wise. Your skin will manufacture vitamin D when it is in contact with the sun.

The recommended daily dose of vitamin D3 for those trying to conceive is 2,000 IU per day (preferably with vitamin K2 as they work as a team for bone health), although testing is advisable as you may need more than this. I took 2,000 – 5,000 iu per day to support my immune system while trying to conceive with regular testing to check my levels.

Vitamin A

Retinoic acid, the metabolite from vitamin A, promotes the induction of T regulatory cells from native T cells, which prevents their conversion into Th17 cells. 'Adequate vitamin A status, whether derived from the ingestion of preformed retinol or beta carotene, is important for maintaining a proper balance of well-regulated T cell functions and for preventing excessive or prolonged inflammatory reactions.' [10]

We can find beta carotene in yellow and orange-coloured fruits and vegetables, as well as leafy green vegetables. We can consume these foods in abundance, eliminating the need to worry about the toxicity associated with excessive intake of the retinol form of vitamin A. Good sources of beta-carotene are carrots, pumpkin, red cabbage, sweet potato, kumara, apricots, mango, cherries, papaya, peaches, watermelon, asparagus, broccoli, Brussel sprouts, kale, lettuce, parsley and spinach. Many of these fruits and vegetables are an excellent source of vitamin C as well, which will provide extra support to the immune system.

Beef liver provides an excellent source of preformed vitamin A (retinol), and you can freeze it raw and grate a small amount into food that is cooking on the stove like a stew or casserole. Other excellent sources of vitamin A are egg yolks, cod liver oil, butter and dairy products.

Reishi mushroom

I have always been very interested in the functional properties of mushrooms, so I took reishi in June 2018 to support my immunity over the winter as I had found reishi to be very effective at providing immune protection for winter ills and chills. It was part of a mushroom blend that included shitake, also known for its immune-modulating and anti-inflammatory properties. This was a month before I conceived my daughter, so I always wondered whether reishi and shitake had played a role in that.

Looking at various studies, a protein found in reishi known as RLZ-8 appears to regulate the Th17/Treg balance by down regulating Th17 cells and upregulating T regulatory cells. In a 2013 study, 'LZ-8 treatment was found to stimulate a 4-fold and 10-fold expansion in the T reg population of murine and human primary CD4 + T Regulatory Cells Respectively.' [11]

If my recurrent chemical pregnancies were because of an imbalance in Th17 and T regulatory cells at the time of implantation, then reishi would have helped to calm down my overactive immune system and stopped it from attacking the fetus, allowing implantation to succeed. If you take reishi while trying to conceive, I recommend that you stop using it once a pregnancy is confirmed because the purpose of using it is to support the immune system during the complexities of the implantation process.

Proteolytic enzymes

Taking proteolytic enzymes for two to four weeks prior to trying to conceive can be a useful way of reducing inflammation and supporting autoimmunity. Proteolytic enzymes are specific enzymes that digest proteins in the body. When taken on an empty stomach away from food, proteolytic enzymes break down and eliminate any problematic proteins in the body. These could be food antigens, blood clots, fibrous tissue, bacteria, yeast and fungi/mould or circulating immune complexes (CICs), which are one of the autoimmune triggers that can cause the body to attack itself.

Circulating immune complexes (CICs) are formed as a result of partially digested protein molecules entering the bloodstream via a leaky gut. These proteins typically come from the incomplete digestion of foods such as wheat, dairy and gluten, because of an impaired digestive system. The weakened intestinal lining (leaky gut) allows these partially digested proteins to be absorbed into the bloodstream, where they circulate. Partially digested proteins are not supposed to be in the bloodstream as they are too large to be metabolised, so the immune system reacts to them as if they are a foreign invader. The immune system produces antibodies, which combine with the proteins to form circulating immune complexes (CICs).

A healthy person can eliminate these circulating immune complexes through their lymphatic system and kidneys. However, an individual with impaired digestion, leaky gut, and multiple food intolerances produces too many CICs that overwhelm the body's ability to eliminate them. `At this point the body has no choice but to store them in its own soft tissues, where the immune system continues to attack them as allergens.' [12]

When the CICs are stored in body tissues, the immune system attacks that tissue (essentially attacking itself), resulting in inflammation and autoimmunity. For example, if the CICs are stored in the thyroid, this may lead to Hashimoto's thyroiditis. If the CICs are stored in the joints, it may lead to rheumatoid arthritis and, if stored in the skin, it may be psoriasis or vitiligo. As the CICs persist and accumulate in various tissues, our chances of developing multiple autoimmune diseases rise. In fact, I have seen clients in my clinic and in the community who have three or four different autoimmune conditions. It is becoming an increasing problem.

When it comes to supporting autoimmunity, we need to get to the root cause of the development of these circulating immune complexes (CICs) by improving digestion, healing and sealing the intestinal lining and eliminating those allergenic foods for a period of time to dampen down the immune response to these foods. Proteolytic enzymes are an important part of this healing process as they gobble up and digest those immune complexes so over time less CICs are stored in body tissues, which results in a reduction of inflammation and risk of autoimmunity.

Proteolytic enzymes are different to digestive enzymes in that they are taking on an empty stomach. If they are taking with food, they would only assist with the digestion of the protein in that meal. When taking on an empty stomach, they have the following benefits:

- Reduces inflammation throughout the body

- Breaking down and removing circulating immune complexes (CICs)

- Dissolves fibrin and clots in the blood, improving blood flow

- Dissolves arterial plaque

- Dissolves scar tissue

- Cleans up the immune system and minimises the impact of allergies

- Cleans the blood of foreign debris

- Kills and eliminates bacteria, virus, fungi and other pathogens

- Breaks down pathogenic biofilms, which is a community of bacteria that colonizes a surface (e.g. the gut lining) and create a complex multicellular matrix (like a protective bubble)

- Reduces the risk of food intolerance reactions

There are several types of proteolytic enzymes that are derived from different sources. A good enzyme formula will have at least 200,000 HUT of protease.

Chapter summary

Silent, low-grade inflammation is exactly that *silent,* so you may not actually know it may be affecting you. If you are experiencing unexplained infertility and recurrent pregnancy loss, think about the symptoms that you have that may contribute to this immune imbalance. This could be joint pain, abdominal gas and bloating, food intolerances, thrush, skin rashes and other allergies, asthma, gut infections, anything really.

The next step would be to work with a naturopath, nutritionist or functional medicine practitioner who can help you get to the root cause of your unexplained infertility and work with you to bring things back into balance with a personalised treatment plan.

Chapter Ten

Recurrent chemical pregnancies

W hen your body keeps saying no, time and time again.

I didn't even know what a chemical pregnancy was until I suffered my first one in 2010, which was when my first son was around 18 months old. When I discovered my period was almost a week late, I wasn't overly excited because I had just started trying to get pregnant again after giving birth to my son in 2008. I guess I didn't quite feel ready to be pregnant again after the trauma of my son's birth, however, after five days of getting used to the idea of being pregnant again, suddenly it was all over as I started bleeding while having morning tea with my son. I was devastated.

It took this unexpected loss to realise that I was actually happy to be pregnant again after all. I then went on a mission to get pregnant as fast as I could. Unfortunately, it took another 10 long years, 17 chemical pregnancies, and two miscarriages later to realise my dream of having a sibling for my son.

Recurrent chemical pregnancies can be a tough road as they occur so early on (between four and five weeks), so they are not technically referred to as normal miscarriages. As a result, you find it harder to seek help from your doctor and fertility specialist. This is because by the time you have sought help, you no longer have a positive pregnancy test or detectable human chorionic gonadotropin (HCG) hormone level in the blood, so there is no actual evidence that you were pregnant.

HCG is a hormone produced by the cells of the placenta during pregnancy. With a later miscarriage, you at least have a record of the HCG test results you get when you first go to the doctor, which is usually around the five-week mark. With chemical pregnancies, it is all over so fast, often before you have had a chance to get any blood tests done.

The more chemical pregnancies I had, the more anxiety I faced toward the end of the two weeks wait. Most months, I just couldn't bring myself to take a home pregnancy test until at least five weeks had passed. Many times, I didn't take a test, but I still knew you just feel different, your body knows.

What are chemical pregnancies?

A chemical pregnancy is a very early miscarriage that occurs when an egg is fertilised but doesn't fully implant in the uterus. The pregnancy is usually over between four and five weeks. If you test early enough, you may have an initial positive pregnancy test, but after a few days, you will likely start to bleed and have a negative pregnancy test as HCG levels drop off. This is referred to as a chemical pregnancy.

Chemical pregnancies are fairly common and if you weren't trying to get pregnant, it would likely feel like a late period that is slightly heavier than normal, so you may not even notice. When you are trying to get pregnant and have a chemical pregnancy, you may feel pregnant during those cycles, so you are more aware that it is happening.

Although I lost count in the end, I estimate that I have suffered about 17 chemical pregnancies over 10 years. I went to my doctor and fertility specialist often to discuss my situation, but they didn't provide me with any useful support as they technically didn't consider them actual miscarriages. They informed me I needed to have at least three "actual miscarriages" before they could refer me for further testing. I did later go on to have two miscarriages at six and eight weeks and had some investigative testing with my fertility clinic. Despite this, my doctor and fertility specialist could not find a reason and labelled me as having unexplained infertility.

My mission at the time was to understand, through research, why I kept having chemical pregnancies repeatedly. After each one, I would try different approaches in terms of diet, lifestyle, and supplements.

Causes of chemical pregnancies

There are many causes of chemical pregnancies, and I explored most of these with myself over the years, but nothing appeared to be obvious. Chemical pregnancies are usually a failure of the embryo to implant properly into the lining of the uterus. It is where an egg becomes fertilised, but the implantation process is not completed. The common causes are:

- Chromosomal abnormalities - around 50%

- Uterine abnormalities, e.g., fibroids, endometriosis

- Gynecological infections

- Low thyroid function

- Hormone imbalances such as a luteal phase defect

- Low body mass index

- Smoking and excessive alcohol consumption

- Autoimmune issues

- Stress

After 10 years of going around and around on this chemical pregnancy roundabout, it surprised me when I conceived naturally at age 43 and gave birth with no complications to a healthy baby girl at age 44. I waited until five and a half weeks to do a pregnancy test as I was expecting the usual chemical pregnancy to occur before five weeks, but amazingly, it didn't. So why, after all this time, did this pregnancy continue? This was purely a miracle. I have identified a couple of key reasons which I think may have contributed to it, but I really don't know for sure.

Even though I had worked on these areas individually over the years, maybe finally everything was in balance and optimally aligned. Or maybe it was just my time. I like to believe this.

Hormones

My cycles were pretty regular, with no PMS, good energy levels, and mood. I had been supporting my progesterone levels for a few months with the herb vitex and homeopathy. I also started taking the mineral boron three months prior to conception as I thought I was experiencing perimenopause and, according to kinesiology testing, I needed this. Revisit chapter six for further information on this. I also lowered my stress levels by reducing my work hours, which made important space for my baby.

Vitamin B12

In chapter 3, I emphasized the importance of vitamin B12 and how vitamin B12 deficiency has been associated with early pregnancy loss, yet doctors rarely test for it. Throughout my journey of 10 years dealing with secondary infertility and recurrent chemical pregnancies, neither my doctor nor fertility clinic mentioned or assessed me for it.

Vitamin B12 ended up being one of my key missing links and when I discovered I was pregnant with my daughter, I took high doses of vitamin B12 during pregnancy in the form of methylcobalamin.

The issue with a B12 deficiency is that it can lead to high levels of homocysteine, especially in people who have MTHFR gene mutations.

What is homocysteine and how does it get elevated?

We produce homocysteine when our body breaks down the amino acid methionine, which is a building block of protein.

Vitamin B12 is part of a family of methyl donors, which includes vitamin B6 and folate that helps your body break down homocysteine and convert it into other amino acids for use by the body.

High levels of homocysteine can occur when there is a deficiency of folate rich foods and foods rich in vitamin B6 and B12 in the diet, so eating these foods can be a great first step.

As a reminder, here are the foods that are rich in each of these methyl donors:

- *Vitamin B12* - Meat, fish, dairy products, eggs

- *Vitamin B6* - Tuna, pork, eggs, banana, liver, salmon, spinach

- *Folate* - Leafy green vegetables, beans, liver, asparagus, eggs

Supplements can help bring down levels of homocysteine, particularly with cases of infertility and recurrent pregnancy loss, when a multivitamin may not be enough. An additional supplement of 500 mcg methylfolate, 1,000 mcg of vitamin B12 as methylcobalamin and 50 mg of vitamin B6 as pyridoxal 5 phosphate, may be effective at bringing down homocysteine levels. Please note that if you have the MTHFR gene mutation or have low levels of vitamin B12 than you may need more than this, so it is best to seek guidance from a qualified practitioner.

Genetic predisposition

Individuals with MTHFR mutations (as discussed in chapter 3) develop elevated homocysteine because they are unable to metabolise folic acid and convert it into methylfolate, so are often folate deficient.

Ovulation and implantation

A deficiency in vitamin B12 can also negatively affect ovulation, impair egg development and quality by disrupting normal cell division, and can contribute to implantation failure. Your doctor can measure homocysteine levels and vitamin B12 by a simple blood test. It may be worth asking for if you feel this could be affecting you.

I optimised folate levels by taking methylfolate and no folic acid at all. For many years, I made the mistake of also taking a prenatal multivitamin with folic acid even though I was taking a separate methylfolate supplement. All folic acid needs to be avoided in favour of methylfolate. Revisit chapter 3 for more information on this.

Immune regulation during the luteal phase and the connection with autoimmunity

I never really knew for certain why I kept having recurrent chemical pregnancies as there was nothing conclusive that came out of any testing I had done. Having said that, I had a gut feeling that there was some immune issue going on which was affecting implantation, as this is the point where everything seemed to fail. I felt it was either an autoimmune issue or an increase in natural killer cells in the uterine lining that essentially attacked the embryo and interfered with implantation. The problem was there was no way of testing this, so I never really knew for sure.

Autoimmune conditions run in my family. My grandmother had autoimmune thyroid disease (as does my aunt), my dad has rheumatoid arthritis, and I found out that I had coeliac disease in my early 30s, and I have been strictly 100% gluten free ever since. My doctor tested me for antinuclear antibodies (ANA), lupus antibodies, and antiphospholipid antibodies twice during my time with my fertility clinic, but there were never any signs of elevated antibodies. This, to me, did not mean that there wasn't an immune reaction going on somewhere, as it is only the presence of many ANA antibodies that show that an autoimmune attack is occurring in the cells and body tissues. I felt I had no problems conceiving, but things went wrong at the implantation stage time and time again.

As I was already strictly 100% gluten free (and I would recommend a gluten free diet for anyone with fertility issues) and I had been working on healing my gut for a long time with periods of time on and off the GAPS Diet, I wondered what else I could do to support my body if there was some sort of immune attack going on. At the time, my health and energy levels were great and previous skin and asthma issues had cleared up. Other than struggling with infertility, I didn't have any health concerns to report.

Supporting autoimmunity with nutrients

The key nutrients to make sure you are optimising if you have an autoimmune condition are vitamin D and selenium, which help to modulate the immune system, so I made sure I took these nutrients each day.

Vitamin D

As discussed in previous chapters, a deficiency in vitamin D has been associated in many studies with recurrent pregnancy loss and unexplained infertility. Supplementing with vitamin D prior to IVF appears to increase the chances of success.

Vitamin D acts as an immune regulator during conception and early pregnancy, so a deficiency can have immunological implications, which may contribute to recurrent pregnancy loss. 'Vitamin D is associated with B and NK cell immunity and Th1/Th2 balance and women with low vitamin D have a tendency to develop APA and other autoantibodies, which are related to autoimmune disease and poor reproductive outcome.'
1

This highlights the need to test for vitamin D as part of a preconception screening programme, although this was not something my fertility doctor ever offered me during my 10-year journey with secondary infertility and recurrent pregnancy loss.

Since I became aware of vitamin D and have taken it regularly, I recognise when I need it the most as my feet would develop a strange tingling sensation when levels were low, and I found taking 2,000 iu when the tingling occurred quickly relieved the symptoms.

When I was pregnant, my feet would tingle like mad, and I found that a combination of vitamin D and magnesium helped to keep my symptoms under control. It was at its worst when I was on a plane ride back from the UK when I was 24 weeks pregnant. I felt that I wanted to cut my feet off and couldn't relax the whole 24-hour flight back, which was torture.

If you are concerned you may be deficient in vitamin D, then you can get a simple blood test done via your doctor, functional medicine practitioner, or naturopath. You can even purchase at-home kits from many pharmacies these days that allow you to do a blood spot test at home.

Optimal levels for a healthy pregnancy are between 30 -40 ng/ML or 75 -100 nmol/L. If you are unsure of your vitamin D levels, it is safe to take 2,000 iu per day as a minimum, especially if you have experienced recurrent pregnancy loss.

Selenium

I thought I had finally solved my infertility issues when I started taking an extra 100 mg of selenium per day back in 2012 and became pregnant a few weeks later. Unfortunately, the pregnancy ended in a miscarriage at seven weeks, but it was the first pregnancy I had that carried on past five weeks, so it was considered an "actual miscarriage" rather than my usual chemical pregnancies. I was devastated when there was no heartbeat at my scans at six and seven weeks and I ended up having to have a dilatation and curettage (D & C) procedure to remove the incomplete miscarriage as my body didn't naturally miscarriage. Despite the trauma of this, a small part of me felt hopeful as I had finally made it past the five-week mark.

Sadly, although the selenium supplement helped, it wasn't the solution, as it took me another seven years to conceive and give birth to my beautiful rainbow baby naturally at age 44.

As I mentioned in chapter 3, having adequate selenium in your diet is important if you have an autoimmune condition such as Hashimoto's thyroiditis, coeliac disease, Crohn's disease, lupus, and psoriasis, as it regulates an excessive immune response and chronic inflammation. Selenium helps to reduce autoantibody levels, so if you have any form of autoimmune condition or are concerned that you may have a hidden autoimmune condition optimising your selenium levels is important.

Dr Isabella Wenz, thyroid pharmacist and author of the book *Hashimoto's Protocol*, recommends the use of around 200 mcg a day to support immune regulation for people with autoimmune conditions. The 100 mcg I took was to top up what I was already taking in my multivitamin, so I was aiming for around 200 mcg a day. It is important not to exceed this level as selenium can be toxic at high levels, so it is always best to work with a qualified practitioner if you are unsure.

Uterine natural killer cells

Natural killer cells (NK) are defined as 'large granular lymphocytes (white blood cells) and are an important component of the innate immune system. Natural killer cells function as one of the first lines of defense, providing protection against viral and bacterial infections and helping to detect and limit the development of cancerous growths.' [2]

Natural killer cells can also be found in the uterine lining, known as CD56 + uterine NK cells, as well as in the blood. 'CD56 uterine natural killer cells are present in human endometrium prior to the initiation of pregnancy and markedly expand to become progressively more granulated during the progesterone dominated secretory phase after ovulation and throughout the first trimester.' [3]

There have been suggestions in early studies that an elevated number of uterine natural killer cells are responsible for early pregnancy loss, as the natural killer cells essentially attack the uterine lining and developing embryo which causes implantation to fail. However, more recent studies have been inconclusive, so it looks like there is still a lot to learn about this subject area. When I was suffering from recurrent chemical pregnancies, the theory of elevated natural killer cells resonated with me, and I continued to investigate it. However, there didn't seem to be anything conclusive in terms of what can be done to reduce these, other than prescribed immunosuppressant medications, which was not an option for me. This is because immunosuppressant drugs are usually only prescribed by fertility doctors if you meet the criteria, which I didn't.

I discovered from my research that some of the biggest factors that lead to an increase in natural killer cells are autoimmune conditions, inflammation, stress, and thyroid imbalances. I always felt that I had these going on under the surface, but not always clear with testing. It is crucial to test for thyroid antibodies to check for autoimmune thyroid issues if you are suffering from recurrent pregnancy loss as this could be what is elevating those natural killer cells. I tried hard to get my thyroid antibodies tested but kept hitting a brick wall as my TSH and free T4 were in the normal range. Luckily, nowadays, you can order your own comprehensive thyroid check through most nutritionists, naturopaths, and functional medicine practitioners. I so wish this was available when I was trying to conceive. It may well have saved me a lot of time and heartache.

Modulating the immune system

As well as taking selenium and vitamin D, I wondered what else I could do naturally to modulate my immune system between conception and implantation to potentially reduce an excess of natural killer cells in my uterine lining if that was what was happening with me.

I tried many things over the years, different supplements, strains of probiotics, and dietary approaches, but nothing really changed until 2018, when I conceived naturally at age 43. This is a summary of what I tried in the six months leading up to when I conceived my daughter, which could have helped to calm down my immune system, allowing the pregnancy to progress:

- *Spore forming probiotics* to regulate the immune system. According to a 2017 study the advantage of a spore forming probiotic over traditional probiotics is that spore forming probiotics are 'composed of endosomes which are highly resistant to acidic pH, are stable at room temperature, and deliver a much greater quantity of high viability bacteria to the small intestines than traditional probiotic supplements.' [4]

- *Vitamin D* as an immune modulator - I needed a therapeutic dose of this daily and I took no less than 2,000 iu per day. I knew when I was low in vitamin D, as my feet would get restless and tingle.

- *Selenium* - I aimed for around 200 mcg a day in total from all sources.

- *Functional mushrooms* - A blend of shitake and reishi mushrooms to help regulate potentially elevated natural killer cells. I took this to support my immune system over the winter.

I took these supplements until I discovered I was pregnant at around five weeks, then stopped the mushrooms but continued with a therapeutic dose of vitamin D, selenium, and probiotics throughout the rest of my pregnancy.

The role of the gut microbiome

The gut microbiome plays a crucial role in modulating the immune system, keeping the two dominant arms of the immune system known as T helper 1 (Th1) and T helper 2 (Th2) in a healthy balance. If the Th1 arm of the immune system becomes more dominant, a person is more prone to autoimmune conditions. If the Th2 arm is more dominant, a person is more prone to allergies such as hay fever and eczema.

Probiotics may help to modulate the two arms of the immune system, especially during the early stages of pregnancy when the immune system is under a lot of stress. Although I don't know exactly why I got pregnant naturally after 10 years of having recurrent chemical pregnancies, one thing I did note is that I switched to taking spore-forming probiotics about three months before I conceived, and I noticed quickly a positive change in my skin health. Since my mid-20s, I have been intermittently struggling with eczema and skin rashes that originated from a two-month antibiotic treatment for persistent folliculitis. I am wondering if the spore-based probiotics successfully restored balance to my immune system, which the other probiotics were unable to do.

Shitake and reishi mushroom for immune modulation

I took a mushroom powder with shitake and reishi to see if this would help modulate my immune system but also to provide general immunity support as we were heading into winter. Reishi mushroom can dampen down an excessive immune response, which is common in autoimmunity, by restoring Th1/Th2 balance. In chapter 9, I discussed how reishi also down regulates Th17 cells and up regulates T regulatory cells, reducing inflammation and calming down an overactive immune response. Reishi also supports the adrenal glands by helping you adapt to the stress going on around you.

Shitake mushroom increases secretory IGA levels and reduces inflammation, so is beneficial for inflammatory conditions such as endometriosis and uterine fibroids. Secretory immunoglobulin IGA is an antibody that protects our mucosal lining from the attack from pathogens and toxins, acting as a first line of defense. Shitake down regulates inflammatory responses and has a beneficial effect on the gut microbiome. I stopped taking it as soon as I found out I was pregnant, but I wonder whether it was enough to keep my immune system from attacking the uterine lining so that implantation could naturally occur, or it helped to reduce my fibroid.

Food intolerances

What we eat plays an important role in the process of implantation, as food can have a direct effect on our immune system, especially if we are eating inflammatory foods or foods that we are intolerant to. Eating foods that cause a reaction can put extra stress on the immune system, which can lead to immune dysregulation. Investigating and eliminating food intolerances is important if you are suffering from recurrent chemical pregnancies and early pregnancy loss, as you ideally want to remove anything that is triggering the immune system. I used to test myself for food sensitivities every few years to see if there was anything putting extra pressure on my immune system.

Inflammation is often to blame

When something goes wrong with the body, inflammation is often to blame. Therefore, it is essential to protect yourself against inflammation by eating plenty of anti-inflammatory foods. The top four foods for reducing inflammation are:

Omega-3

Foods such as salmon, tuna, mackerel, cod liver oil, flaxseed oil, hempseed oil, chia seeds and walnuts are rich in omega-3, which are anti-inflammatory.

Turmeric

The active compound curcumin in turmeric has potent anti-inflammatory action. You can use more turmeric in cooking such as curries and spicy soups, but I would recommend that you also add some black pepper and a source of fat as this increases the bioavailability of the turmeric.

Berries

Brightly coloured berries such as strawberries, blueberries, and blackberries have potent antioxidant and anti-inflammatory action.

Leafy green vegetables

Spinach, kale, silver beet, rocket and mesclun are all rich in nutrients and antioxidants that help to reduce inflammation.

Chapter summary

In summary, recurrent chemical pregnancies can be a very frustrating and lonely journey with very little support from medical specialists, as it is all over so early and hard to prove. If you are suffering from recurrent chemical pregnancies as I did, I would recommend considering the following options:

- Ask your doctor to test for autoimmune diseases. Make sure to request the antinuclear antibodies (ANA) test if you haven't already, to check for elevated autoantibodies attacking your body tissues. It is also important to get screened for antiphospholipid antibodies (APA) to see if blood clotting is an issue.

- If you feel you are reacting to foods, work with a qualified practitioner who can organise food intolerance testing for you or can guide you safely through an elimination protocol. Food intolerance reactions can trigger the immune system and cause inflammation.

- Support your gut health with a spore-based probiotic.

- Look at taking vitamin D and selenium to modulate the immune system.

- Support healthy methylation with methylfolate and look at getting your B12 checked to see if you need this as well. See chapter 3 for more information on folate.

- Consider functional mushrooms like reishi and shitake for immune modulation if needed.

- Reduce inflammation with omega-3 essential fatty acids, turmeric, berries and leafy green vegetables.

- Support stress levels with deep breathing, meditation, and fertility yoga. See chapter 7 for more on stress and adrenal support.

Chapter Eleven

Male factor infertility

I nfertility can affect both men and women, but very often the focus is on the female, which is understandable as they will grow and carry the baby. However, we must not forget that 50% of a child's DNA comes from the male, so it is essential that future dads-to-be prioritise their health as well.

The statistics on the worldwide decline in sperm health are alarming and I am seeing more and more men book in to see me in my clinic with low sperm count, poor motility and abnormal morphology, which is the form, shape and structure. They are often completely surprised when they receive the results of their semen analysis.

'Sperm counts around the world have halved over the past 50 years, with the pace of decline more than doubling since 2000.' [1] A 2019 journal also highlights that 'sperm concentration, morphology and semen volume have all been shown to deteriorate drastically over the past decade.' [2]

There are many factors that can affect the health of sperm. The most common ones are smoking, excessive alcohol, radiation, exposure to toxins, getting overheated, poor diet, inflammation, infections, nutritional deficiencies, hormone imbalances and a varicocele, which is an enlarged vein in the scrotum. Studies have shown that 'smokers could increase DNA fragmentation by an average of 9.19 per cent compared to non-smokers. Also, air pollution, exposure to pesticides and insecticides increased sperm DNA fragmentation by an average of 9.68 per cent.' [3]

Advancing age is also an overlooked factor for men with 'the decrease in sperm fertilisation rate starting between the ages of 45 and 50 years.' [4]

Toxins are everywhere, pesticides and toxic chemicals are in our homes, in our gardens and in our food supply, which has contributed to a worldwide decline in sperm health. Yet despite the many known factors contributing to reduced sperm health, approximately 30–40 % of male infertility cases are still unexplained.

DNA damage to sperm can not only cause infertility, but it can also increase the risk of miscarriage and could lead to birth defects. It is important to educate our dads-to-be on the diet, lifestyle, and environmental factors that can damage sperm. For example, how many men do you know that walk around with a mobile phone in their front pocket? or sit with an iPad on their lap for hours a day? This can be a direct source of radiation that can damage sperm.

Three months before you start trying to conceive is when your health should be at its most optimal. This is because it takes approximately 100 days for new sperm to be produced. This means that your sperm now reflects how healthy you have been over the last three months.

So, what can you do to optimise the health of your sperm in the three-month preconception period?

Nutrition

To improve sperm health nourishment is the key and therefore your diet needs to be nutrient dense and rich in antioxidants. You can achieve this by consuming at least five servings of vegetables a day and two servings of fruit.

Where possible and affordable, choose organic fruit and vegetables to reduce exposure to pesticides and herbicides, which can affect sperm health. Ensure you have at least one serving a day of leafy greens such as kale, mesclun, and spinach for active folate to support methylation and optimal cell health. When choosing vegetables, opt for a rainbow of bright colours for antioxidants.

Commit to eating a whole foods diet, with limited processed foods and refined sugar. Limit packet foods like biscuits, cakes, pies, and crackers. Choose food you can make at home from scratch.

A good general rule is to have a source of healthy fat and protein with each meal. Good examples of healthy fats are organic butter, coconut oil, eggs, avocado, bone broth, meat stock, fish, and nuts. Fat is a building block to make hormones, transports cholesterol and helps to reduce inflammation. For protein, choose grass-fed meat, organic chicken, organic dairy products (e.g., kefir, yoghurt, cheese, milk) organic eggs, fish, shellfish, nuts, seeds, beans and legumes. Protein is the building blocks of body cells and tissues and provides amino acids essential for sperm production and healthy hormones.

Key nutrients that support sperm health

Nutritional deficiencies can also contribute to poor sperm health and can be a consequence of a diet lacking in nutrient-dense foods, soils lacking minerals, and poor gut health affecting absorption. Here are the key nutrients to optimise with diet and supplements where needed.

Zinc

The trace mineral zinc is essential for improving the quality, quantity, and motility of sperm. It is also a key mineral for immune health, reducing anti-sperm antibodies, and increasing testosterone levels (more on this later in this chapter). Experts recommend a daily supplement dose of at least 30 mg zinc, preferably with a small dose of copper, to maintain a healthy balance of zinc and copper levels. This is because zinc and copper are antagonistic minerals, and excessive zinc intake can deplete copper levels. To increase zinc levels with food, add a tablespoon of pumpkin seeds to smoothies or breakfast cereals. Oysters, eggs, meat, poultry, nuts, seafood, and dairy are all excellent sources.

Selenium

A common deficiency in men is selenium, as it is a mineral that is lacking in our soils. Selenium is vital for sperm count, morphology (shape and structure), and motility. Selenium is also an important antioxidant that helps to prevent DNA fragmentation. Aim for around 150–200 mcg a day from all supplement sources. It is important to avoid exceeding 200 mcg per day unless a qualified practitioner guides you, as higher amounts may be toxic when taken long term. Good food choices are Brazil nuts, fish, poultry, whole grains, and eggs.

Omega-3 essential fatty acids

Studies have shown that omega-3 essential fatty acids improve sperm quality, reduce inflammation, and decrease DNA damage. Aim to have oily fish such as tuna, salmon, sardines, and mackerel at least two to three times a week for an excellent source of omega-3 essential fatty acids. Also, flaxseed oil, hemp seed oil, walnuts, and chia seeds are rich in omega-3. You may need to supplement with omega-3 if you do not feel you are getting enough in your diet.

Coenzyme Q10

Supplementing with coenzyme Q10 for at least three months leading up to IVF treatment has a lot of research supporting its effectiveness in optimising sperm health. It increases sperm count, motility, morphology, and its overall vitality. The other benefits of coenzyme Q10 are that it supports mitochondrial health and energy production and is an antioxidant that helps to combat oxidative stress by fighting free radical damage. The general recommendation is to take 200 mg a day of coenzyme Q10 as ubiquinol, which is the better absorbed form. In severe cases of low sperm count, taking 400 mg daily is even more beneficial. A 2019 study reported that 'coenzyme Q10 improved sperm motility, concentration, and semen antioxidant status in infertile men, with a greater improvement observed in response to a dose of 400 mg a day than a dose of 200mg a day.' [5] You could just take 400 mg a day for an enhanced response, but if cost is a factor, 200 mg is still beneficial.

Vitamin C

The superstar nutrient vitamin C is also an important antioxidant for increasing sperm count, motility, and morphology. Vitamin C helps to prevent sperm from clumping together, therefore improving its ability to swim. Citrus fruits, berries, pepper, kiwi, broccoli, Brussel sprouts, potatoes, and tomatoes are all excellent sources of vitamin C. You may also want to consider supplementing with liposomal vitamin C, which is gentle but well absorbed.

L-carnitine

The amino acid derivative and antioxidant l-carnitine has also shown in studies to be beneficial for improving sperm health. As an antioxidant, it helps to protect sperm against the excessive production of free radicals that might lead to sperm damage. Research suggests that l-carnitine increases sperm motility, improved sperm concentration and morphology. ' [6]

According to a recent study in 2023, 'overall evidence supports that l-carnitine can positively impact male fertility, even at relatively low doses of 2 g per day. This supplement enhances sperm parameters, regulates hormone levels, reduces ROS (reactive oxygen species) levels and subsequently improves fertility rates.' [7]

You can optimise l-carnitine levels by eating protein-rich foods such as red meat, poultry, fish, and dairy foods. Vegetables, fruit, and grains have small amounts. L-carnitine is also available as a supplement in most health shops and the recommended dose is 2 g per day. Most supplements contain 50 mg capsules, so this would be four capsules a day.

Additional support

Alcohol

It would be worth reducing your alcohol intake as alcohol increases oxidative stress in the body and, several studies have found that regular alcohol consumption decreases sperm count, motility, and fertilisation rates. Stick to a couple of drinks at weekends. If you need a refreshing drink during the week (that is also good for your gut and therefore good for your health overall) choose kombucha, or sparkling water with lime or lemon. You could also try it with or one or two tablespoons of apple cider vinegar, which I think tastes similar to cider.

Gut health

We now know that whatever is happening in your gut will be affecting the rest of your body, and sperm health is no exception. According to Dr Natasha Campbell McBride, author of *Gut and Physiology Syndrome* 'our health very much depends on the health of our gut flora. No matter how far from the gut an organ of your body is, it is greatly affected by the gut flora's composition, state, and function.' [8]

Improving your gut health should be a priority. A properly functioning digestive system breaks down food, absorbs nutrients, and removes toxins that can affect fertility. A healthy digestive system ensures you are absorbing crucial nutrients for reproductive health. Even if you have a very healthy diet, if you are not absorbing the nutrients from your food properly, you will have nutritional deficiencies which can lead to mineral imbalances and hormone imbalances.

Unlike studies on female fertility, there is limited research on the effects of gluten on sperm health. However, anything that is causing inflammation in your gut will be affecting your whole body and increasing oxidative stress. As it takes approximately 100 days for new sperm to be produced, it would be worth eliminating gluten for at least three months if you have been struggling with infertility for a while and your semen analysis is less than optimal.

Environmental factors

Reduce your exposure to environmental toxins by using natural skin care and cleaning products, drinking filtered water and avoid using plastic drink bottles and plastic containers and never use them in the microwave.

Keep your distance from your cell phones, as keeping a cell phone in your pocket can expose sperm to radiation, which can negatively affect sperm health. Also, avoid using an iPad or laptop on your lap.

Stay as cool as possible as elevated temperatures can impair sperm quality. Try to avoid taking hot baths or showers and wearing tight fitted underwear. Staying cool is extremely important if you have a varicocele, which is a common condition that affects about 15% of men and causes the veins in the scrotum to enlarge. Fertility experts believe that the enlarged veins contribute to infertility by raising the temperature in the scrotum and decreasing sperm production.

Ensure you are hydrated as dehydration essentially dries up sperm making motility difficult. Aim for 30 mls of water for each KG of body weight. On a day when you do cardio exercise, especially in hot weather, aim for an additional 500 mls – 1 litre.

Low testosterone

Another factor to consider with male infertility is whether low testosterone levels, known as hypogonadism, may be reducing sperm count and making it difficult to conceive.

Many men don't have optimal testosterone levels because of stress, inflammation, a poor diet, smoking, alcohol, and exposure to toxins. Here are some of the common symptoms of low testosterone in men, could this be affecting you?

- Reduced libido and erectile function

- Low sperm count

- Fatigue and exhaustion

- Loss of body hair on face and body

- Obesity

- Loss of lean muscle mass

- Depression, anxiety, insomnia.

Here are some strategies which may help increase testosterone levels naturally.

Zinc

The fact that I am talking about zinc again shows how important it is for male fertility. Zinc is involved as a cofactor in over 300 enzyme functions in the body. It is also one of the trace minerals that is depleted by stress. As well as everything else going on in our lives, infertility is stress, chronic stress, so if our zinc stores get depleted, that is over 300 metabolic functions in the body that will be affected!

Zinc helps to regulate hormones and increase testosterone levels. Zinc-rich foods are oysters, beef, lamb, pumpkin seeds, lentils, mushrooms, spinach, and avocado. Supplementing with extra zinc may be beneficial if you are not getting enough dietary zinc, have an underactive thyroid or you are under a lot of stress.

Dietary fats

The body uses dietary cholesterol to produce testosterone. If you are not eating enough fat, or you do not absorb fat that well because of digestive issues, then the body may not have adequate cholesterol to make hormones. Aim to have a serving of healthy fats with each meal. This may include meat fat, butter, cheese, fermented dairy, sour cream, coconut oil, meat stock, avocado, salmon, nuts, seeds, and olive oil.

Magnesium

Researchers have found a correlation between low magnesium levels and low testosterone levels, and that supplementing with magnesium can restore levels to within normal ranges. Magnesium is another mineral that is depleted by stress and is a cofactor in over 300 metabolic functions of the body. Magnesium-rich foods include almonds, cashews, seeds, bananas, avocados, brown rice, and leafy green vegetables.

It is challenging to get enough magnesium from food, so taking an additional magnesium supplement may help to lower the stress hormone cortisol, which will have a knock-on effect of increasing DHEA and testosterone levels as stress and high cortisol levels deplete them.

Magnesium also inhibits testosterone from binding to sex hormone binding globulin (SHBG) which reduces the free testosterone available for use. My preference is to use a supplement with magnesium glycinate as it is better absorbed and can be helpful for sleep issues.

Weight bearing exercise

Try to do some resistance training with some weights at least three times a week, as this can help to increase testosterone levels naturally. This can also include exercises that use your own body weight, such as squats, lunges and planks. Brief bursts of high-interval training like sprints, star jumps, etc. can also increase testosterone levels.

Chapter summary

To sum up, if your sperm analysis is less than optimal, try not to despair. There are several steps you can take to boost the health and vitality of your sperm. Here are some actions you can take:

- Eat a nutrient-dense diet rich in antioxidants. Aim for a rainbow a day of five brightly coloured vegetables and two fruits. At least one should be leafy green vegetables for a rich form of folate. Choose organic where possible and affordable.

- Optimise the key nutrients that support sperm health and testosterone production through food choices and supplements: these are zinc, selenium, omega-3, coenzyme Q10, Vitamin C, magnesium, and l-carnitine.

- Reduce or eliminate alcohol and smoking as excessive intake causes oxidative stress, which can increase the risk of DNA damage to the sperm.

- Reduce your exposure to environmental toxins by choosing natural skin care and cleaning products and avoid using plastic drink bottles and containers.

- Keep your cell phone out of your pocket and use a laptop or iPad at a desk rather than on your lap. This is to reduce exposure to radiation.

- Keep as cool as possible by avoiding hot baths, showers or hot tubs and wear loose fitted underwear. This is especially important if you have a varicocele.

Chapter Twelve

Listen to your body

We are all unique. There is no one way of eating or supplement plan that is suitable for everyone. This is especially true with infertility.

One of the most important things I did during my fertility journey was to take the time to listen to my body and what it needed. I achieved this through meditation, regularly asking the universe for guidance and through kinesiology, which is also known as muscle testing. According to the Kinesiology Association, a UK registered charity, kinesiology is a holistic therapy that tests muscle response to determine imbalances and can be used to help choose methods to rebalance the body. This technique involves applying pressure to a muscle in the body, typically the fingers or an arm, to assess its strength (a kinesiologist usually does this, but you can also learn to test yourself). They then test the muscle again while you are holding a food or supplement in the other hand. If the food or supplement weakens the muscle, then the food or supplement is thought to have a negative effect on the body. If, on the other hand, the muscle remains strong this is a positive reaction indicating that the food or supplement is beneficial.

In the first few years of my 10-year infertility journey, I spent a lot of time searching the internet for advice in fertility forums. I would often try out expensive supplements just because it worked for someone on a forum or research said it was good for fertility. I achieved very little success in doing this and soon turned inward for answers instead.

While I was working at a health shop in Mount Maunganui in New Zealand, I worked alongside this amazing naturopath who was also a very experienced kinesiologist. She would use muscle testing to get answers from clients about what they needed in terms of supplements and dosages. She would often practice on me in between customers, and I found it fascinating to watch what she came up with. I was so inspired by this that I attended a couple of training courses on muscle testing techniques. I attended a three-day course from Biotrace on Quantum Reflex Analysis and a weekend attending a Touch for Health Kinesiology level 1 course, both in New Zealand. I learned the "O-ring" technique, where you use your hands to test the reaction of a muscle, along with other more advanced muscle testing techniques. After I became more confident with muscle testing, I started practicing the techniques on my clients to test the suitability of products.

After a lot of practice, I could use muscle testing to determine whether I needed to take a supplement or not. I actually became a little obsessed and would go through my pantry, testing all my supplements to see what I needed to take that day. I understood that taking a supplement that my body didn't need, even if it was recommended, wouldn't provide any benefits. This was the approach I took during the last couple of years before I conceived and throughout my pregnancy, and I gained some really valuable insight about my body. There were supplements that tested positive as everyday essentials. These were omega-3, folate, vitamin D, a probiotic, vitamin B12, my prenatal multivitamin and others that I needed less often.

As well as looking at supplements, I also used muscle testing to determine if any foods were potentially triggering my immune system and causing a reaction. It would appear my body was not happy with A1 milk at all, even in small amounts. This was probably because of my history of asthma and the reactivity of the beta casein protein in A1 milk, which can cause sensitivities. Switching to A2 milk really made a difference.

You can also use a pendulum to seek answers from yourself, and you can easily buy one from most crystal retailers. Go to a crystal shop and purchase a pendulum that really speaks to you with its attractiveness and energy. Cleanse the crystal by running it under water for a few minutes to clear any previous negative energies that the crystal has absorbed. Set your intention for the crystal pendulum by saying to it, "I am open to receiving guidance about what I need".

Hold the pendulum with one hand, so it dangles over a table or flat surface. Ask it a question and watch if it starts to spin around in a circle or up and down. If it is not moving, you can give it a little nudge to get it going but try not to force it to swing. Get familiar with the crystal pendulum by asking it to "show my yes" or "show me no" as you hold it. Once you have got the hang of it, you can use it to test supplements or foods by holding it over the top of the item and watching which way it swings. If it swings around in a circle, that was my yes, with up and down for no. Why don't you give this a try as a way of listening to your body?

Crystals for support

As well as a pendulum, I also had a team of crystals that I would call on for support when I needed it. I would carry them around in my pocket, wear them in my bra, or hold them during meditation. Many crystals have energetic healing properties, whether emotional or physical, that are helpful to support fertility and balance hormones.

Each crystal has its own electromagnetic healing energy which, when held or worn close to the body, can influence the body to heal any energy related imbalances.

While there are no scientific studies on the use of crystals for fertility, that doesn't mean you can't have positive results from using them. If they make you feel better emotionally and physically, then there is absolutely a benefit in using them.

Below, I summarise the key crystals in my support crew. I would muscle test each crystal every day to decide whether I should wear or hold it. That is how obsessed I became!

Rose quartz

According to Judy Hall in her book *The Crystal Bible, A Definitive Guide to Crystals,* 'Rose quartz is the stone of unconditional love and infinite peace. It is the most important crystal for the heart and the heart chakra, teaching the true essence of love. It purifies and opens the heart at all levels and brings deep inner healing and self-love. It is calming, reassuring and excellent for a trauma or crisis.' [1]

As the crystal of universal love, rose quartz is rich in healing properties and surrounds you with love and compassion. It promotes inner peace and provides emotional protection.

Rose quartz was my support after my many chemical pregnancies and miscarriages. I would hold a palm sized rose quartz in my hand when I felt upset and it felt like a warm hug, like someone holding your hand. I also wore a small rose quartz in my bra for weeks afterwards, which made me feel supported in a little way.

Moonstone

Known as the crystal of feminine energy, moonstone has a connection to the moon and to intuition. Moonstone can influence the female reproductive cycle and balance hormones. 'Physically moonstone powerfully affects the female reproductive cycle and eases menstrual related disease and tension. It is linked to the pineal gland and balances the hormonal system, stabilising fluid imbalances and attunes to the biorhythmic clock.' [2]

I kept a moonstone on my bedside table so that I could absorb the healing frequencies throughout the night. I had heard that it was best not to wear moonstone during a full moon, as it can be especially powerful and may encourage lucid dreams, so I was reluctant to wear it all the time.

Carnelian

A crystal of life force and vitality, carnelian activates the base chakra, which is the energy centre of the reproductive organs. It can dissolve any energetic blocks and help with any reproductive challenges.

I often would lie with a carnelian over my uterus and meditate, while visualising my child to be. I also wore it alongside other crystals in my bra, as it has a cleansing effect on other stones, cleansing them of any negative energies.

Green aventurine

I have a beautiful green aventurine that is shaped like a large teardrop. It is recognised as one of the top crystals for enhancing fertility.

Green aventurine encourages a sense of optimism and self-confidence and helps to ease worries about the future. It helps to increase energy and brings peace, harmony, and luck.

To be open to receiving good fortune and prosperity, hold a green aventurine in your left hand while meditating. Aim to sit in silence, holding this crystal and focusing on your breathing for at least five minutes a day.

Lepidolite

If you struggle with anxiety, lepidolite is a crystal that promotes peace and serenity. During the two week wait, I would hold a flat, palm-sized lepidolite in my hand to ease my anxiety. The large flat stone felt like someone was holding my hand and reassuring me.

Clear quartz

Clear quartz is the crystal for achieving dreams. You can meditate with clear quartz to gain clarity and amplify your intentions. I often held a clear quartz in my left-hand during meditation, which is the hand for receiving (the right hand is for giving). It was my way of letting the universe know I was ready to receive the gift of a pregnancy and that this was my dream.

Amethyst

The popular crystal amethyst is a great crystal to wear or keep on your bedside table during the two week wait, or all the time if you need it. It helps to balance emotions, especially when you are feeling overwhelmed and stressed, which is often the case when you are coping with the ups and downs of infertility. It also helps to provide support when you are feeling sadness and grief, which is why I often wore it after experiencing a pregnancy loss.

Smoky quartz

Another member of the quartz family, smoky quartz is a protective stone that is grounding and helps to stabilise emotions. It is thought to help increase fertility by having a positive and stimulating effect on the reproductive organs and clearing blockages. It is great to hold in your hand during meditation or to wear close to your body.

So why not try getting hold of some of these crystals to help with your own fertility journey? There may not be much scientific data around to prove that they influence fertility, but to me, crystals were a welcome addition to my fertility toolbox. If they make you feel better and offer you some support and hope, then go for it.

Should you give up?

"The moment you are ready to quit is usually the moment right before the miracle happens. Please don't give up" - unknown.

Many times, during my 10-year journey with secondary infertility, I wanted to give up, but I never totally did. This quote was one reason, as every time I saw it, it inspired me to keep going despite the odds being stacked against me. I wrote the quote on the inside of my diary so I would see it often. What if I quit now, right before the miracle was about to happen? It would be a waste of 10 years working towards this goal. I had to believe that the miracle could still happen, although it seemed so unlikely at the time. Anyone who has been on a long infertility journey will know that you can't just switch off and stop trying, even if you wanted to. There's always a "what if" in the back of your mind.

My situation is living proof that miracles can happen:

- It took me 10 years of trying to conceive with no success. I experienced multiple chemical pregnancies, miscarriages, and an unsuccessful IVF attempt.

- At 39, my AMH test came back very low in the red zone, indicating poor egg reserve.

- After my failed IVF at age 41, I was told by my fertility specialist that I was too old to get pregnant and that my only hope was to use donor eggs

The odds of getting pregnant was very bleak for my age group. If you are over the age of 40, you statistically have:

- A 33% chance of miscarriage, which increases to 50% over age 45

- Less than 5% chance of getting pregnant each month

- An average of about 10% genetically normal eggs

Despite this, I conceived a healthy baby girl naturally at age 43 with no medical intervention and gave birth when I was 44.

Miracles may happen to you too, so try not to give up hope, as success may be just around the corner. I always had this gut feeling that I would eventually get pregnant. It was a feeling or knowing that I just couldn't shift, even when things were not looking hopeful for us at all. I truly believed that my recurrent chemical pregnancies and miscarriages were simply a sign that it wasn't my time, and the universe had a better plan for me. When I got pregnant at age 43, I was in a much better space than I had been previously. I had quit my 30 hours a week job at a health shop that was dragging me down and for the first time in 10 years, I truly had the space mentally and physically for the baby. My stress levels were reduced, I was no longer handling till receipts each day at work (which are coated with hormone disruptive chemicals) and I had more time to focus on just me and my business. Amazingly, three weeks after quitting my job at the health shop, I discovered I was pregnant naturally.

Telling the universe about your baby dreams

"What you seek is seeking you," Rumi

If you are currently trying to get pregnant, have you actually taken the time to write down your goals to let the universe know how much you desire a baby? This was something I did consistently during the last three years of my 10-year fertility journey and I like to believe it made a difference although it is hard to know for sure.

Every Monday, I would take myself to a cafe to write about my life and business goals for the week and month. Each week I would write something like:

"I would love very much to get pregnant and carry my beautiful child to full term if it is safe for me to do so. I am so grateful. Please show me signs of what I need to do to achieve this."

During my meditation practice, I would start by reminding myself of my goal. Throughout the following week, I would pay attention to any potential signs from the universe, like coming across a social media post, a supplement falling off a shelf at work, or a sudden thought that enters my mind.

It took a few years of consistently writing my goals down weekly to the universe before my baby dream finally came into reality. I felt that each sign I listened to or change I made brought me closer to my goal.

So, I encourage you to purchase one of those attractive sparkly notepads and write down your goal of having a baby weekly to the universe. Write how grateful you are and that you are very open to receiving signs from the universe of what you need to do to work towards your goal. You can even go as far as to describe your baby in terms of what he or she will look like and his or her name if you have thought that far ahead. I often wrote about my beautiful baby girl Jenah. Even as I approached my mid-40s, I always had a feeling that I would eventually have a baby girl, and this would be her name. I never gave up hope.

Surrender to the universe

The concept of surrendering to the universe is something I learned from Gabby Bernstein, author of the book *Super Attractor*. In her book, she writes that sometimes you need to let go of trying to control things and surrender to the universe. Trust that the universe has a plan for you. This gave me hope that I would get pregnant when it was the right time for the greater good of the universe. I tried to adopt this mindset mentally instead of being impatient about wanting to get pregnant as soon as possible, or when I thought it was a good time for me.

"When you face challenges, know that there is a plan beyond your own"
Gabby Bernstein.

Looking back, there was no better time to have a baby than when Jenah was born. My son was older and more self-sufficient, I was no longer studying, and I had quit my 30-hour a week retail job that was draining my energy. I was also feeling hopeful about the future as I was working on a plan to build my business. I was focusing on the positives of my life rather than the negatives.

I finally felt that I had space in my life to have a baby. Although I desperately wanted another baby for almost 10 years and tried everything to have one, there really was no better time than when Jenah was born. It felt that everything was finally in alignment.

Positive affirmations

I would often use positive affirmations to help with my mindset, especially during the two week wait when I often found myself crippled with anxiety. My feelings of anxiety would get worse in the few days leading up to when my period was due.

Affirmations are positive statements that are used to challenge negative or unhelpful thought patterns. Repeating positive affirmations can help to overcome negativity, build self-confidence, and view situations in a more positive light. Aimee Raupp talks about the connection between the brain and the rest of the body in her book *Body Belief* and quotes throughout the book

"The body hears what the brain says"

I had a little red notepad by my bed and every night I would read my positive affirmations to myself. It is important to commit to repeating your affirmations daily as the more you repeat them, the stronger your beliefs will lead to positive changes. Here were some of my affirmations:

- I am in perfect health, physically, mentally, emotionally, and spiritually, to conceive my child

- Everything that is happening to me now is happening to me for my ultimate good

- I am happy, healthy, and ready to conceive my baby

- I fully accept myself, no matter what

- I am strong and my body is open to new life

- My uterus is a healthy place to nourish my baby

- I am looking forward to meeting my beautiful, healthy child

- I am grateful for my body and what it is capable of

- I am the best version of myself

- I dream, I believe, I receive

Now choose some positive affirmations that really speak to you and write them down in a place that will allow you to see them often. This could be in your diary, in a notepad or post it notes on your wall. It doesn't matter where you write them, as long as you see them regularly and speak the words to yourself daily. Positive affirmations need to be in the present tense and not related to the past or present. This allows you to be more mindful, living in the moment and not worrying about the past or future.

What do you believe about your health?

In the *Oxford Dictionary,* the definition of a belief is an 'acceptance that something exists or is true, especially one without proof.' It is something that you believe or accept as truth based on a fact, opinion, or assumption.

Do you truly believe that you can get pregnant? When I was in the thick of my infertility journey, on some days I strongly believed that I couldn't hold on to pregnancies and this became my narrative. In my mind, it was the reason I kept having chemical pregnancies and recurrent miscarriages. Looking back, I realise now that this narrative I kept telling myself was likely telling the rest of my body that I couldn't hold on to a pregnancy. A few questions to ask yourself:

- What are your beliefs?

- Do you feel your body is capable of getting pregnant?

- Are you living with the label of infertility, endometriosis, thyroid issues, PCOS?

- What affirmations can you repeat daily to help change the belief in your mind that you have a health problem that is holding you back?

The two-week wait

It is impossible to write a book about secondary infertility without mentioning the dreaded two-week wait, the time of the month that can be the most frustrating and confusing.

The dreaded two-week wait is the time of the month from just after ovulation until you either find out you are pregnant, or your period arrives. Only people who have been actively trying to conceive would know the term "two-week wait" as it is often talked about in online fertility forums. It is a very stressful time for many, especially for those who are going through IVF, and they have their pregnancy test date looming.

The two-week wait can be an exciting and hopeful time as there is a chance you may actually be pregnant and some days you really do feel pregnant. It is also a very stressful time, full of nervousness and anticipation, especially in the few days before your period is due. What makes the long-term infertility rollercoaster so tough to bear is the up and down emotions you experience throughout the monthly cycle. If your cycle is anything like mine, it would go like this.

Day 1 – 5

My period arrives, and I am absolutely devastated for two days. Over these first few days of my cycle, I would grieve that there is no baby and my fertility diet would totally go out the window. This is a time for having a few alcoholic drinks and eating all those naughty foods that are not advisable to eat if you were pregnant, think lots of wine, coffee, and chocolate.

Day 5 – 10

My heart has started to heal, and I feel a bit more optimistic again. I look ahead to this cycle and to ovulation which is approaching. I focus on what I can do differently this cycle to increase my chances, whether a new supplement, meditation app, or lifestyle change.

Day 10 – 15

This is the business end of the cycle where all the focus is on "baby dancing" as they call it in the forums and doing everything you can to maximise your chances of conceiving.

Day 15 – 21

This is the week after ovulation till the time when implantation is likely to occur. This stage is where you can relax for a bit and know that the work is done for the month as it is too early for symptoms and to take a pregnancy test. A time to distract yourself with other non-fertility related activities to help pass the time and to have a brief break from it all.

Day 21 – 28 (If you have a 28-day cycle)

This is the point where you may get the odd twinge or unusual symptom that could be either a sign of early pregnancy or bad PMS. The symptoms are so similar it is hard to know the difference, and it is challenging not to overthink things and be too hopeful. I would experience dragging in my uterus, sore breasts, sore back, and a feeling that something was going on inside. When this happened, I convinced myself I was pregnant and would obsess over every symptom I had. I became increasingly anxious after day 26, fearing the presence of blood every time I went to the toilet.

Day 28

It is test day if you have a regular 28-day cycle and you haven't already had to take a pregnancy test earlier as a part of an IVF procedure. This is the earliest I would take a pregnancy test. Some months, though, I was too scared to take a test for the fear of it being negative that I would leave it until about five weeks before testing. Very often I was about five days late and I would take a test only to get a period just before. It scared me to test because I had chemical pregnancies so often. When my period did eventually arrive, as it did for 10 years, I was again back to the despair and devastation, a chance to grieve and heal before the next cycle.

As the years went on, I felt numb rather than grief whenever my period arrived. I really believed this was my body's protective mechanism kicking in to guard me from the ongoing unbearable stress and upset. If this is true, it really is amazing what the body can do.

Coping activities

I developed my own coping activities to help reduce stress and to act as a distraction during the two-week wait. These were:

- To start reading an interesting new fiction book right after ovulation. It kept me from wasting time searching for pregnancy symptoms online. It needs to be a book that really captures your attention, so you look forward to reading it. My books of choice were the *Outlander* series by Diana Gabaldon, and I worked my way through all eight of her large novels during my infertility journey.

- If there is a best time to do meditation, then the two-week wait is the time. Every day, I allocated at least 10 minutes to meditate using the apps *Headspace* and *Smiling Minds*. I felt that this really helped to calm down my overthinking mind and think more positively.

- I finished each day with four restorative yoga poses. These are simple yoga poses that you hold for a longer period than traditional poses, which helps to relax you, reduce stress, improves circulation and promotes sleep. The poses I would typically use are legs up the wall, child's pose, butterfly pose, wide leg forward fold and seated twists.

- Fill your time with household chores that you have been putting off and listen to a captivating audiobook or podcast while you clean to help pass the time.

- Get out in nature with daily walks. This is one of the best ways to clear your mind. If you live near the beach, take a walk barefoot along the sand to experience the energetic benefits of grounding.

- Schedule time to chat online to others via fertility forums to find support with people who are on the same journey as you. Try to limit this time though, as spending too much time in this environment can actually increase your anxiety. Often, the information given out in forms is unreliable, especially regarding supplements.

- It is hard not to overanalyse every twinge in the body and feel convinced you are pregnant. This happened to me so often and most of the time I ended up getting my period, so obviously I wasn't pregnant. Try to tell yourself that feeling pregnant doesn't always mean you are actually pregnant, as very often PMS symptoms are very similar to early pregnancy symptoms. My mind seemed to be much more alert to these symptoms in the two-week wait.

- Try not to take a pregnancy test until your period is due. This is especially important if you suffer from frequent early chemical pregnancies like I did. If the pregnancy is going to end just after four weeks, it may be easier if you didn't know you were actually pregnant, as there is nothing more heartbreaking than seeing a faint positive test result and getting your period a few days later. When you see the test result, although faint, it gives you so much hope and happiness only to have that ripped away from you a few days later. I always tested at about five weeks for this exact reason, to protect myself from further heartbreak. I was also too stressed and anxious to even consider testing earlier than this. When I had my only IVF cycle, they organised a test on day 10 after egg transfer and my god, the stress was unbearable. I had to take the blood test at 9 am at the hospital and wait for a phone call from the nurse that afternoon. I couldn't concentrate on anything that day, as I was so stressed and anxious. The phone call was good news though as I received the news that I was pregnant with a healthy level of HCG hormone. Unfortunately, this was short-lived as I ended up having an early miscarriage at about six weeks.

- Practice deep breathing to calm the body and mind. Take a deep breath in slowly to the count of four. Hold for four seconds, then breathe out slowly to the count of seven. Try to do this at least five times in one session. This will help calm your nervous system.

- The second week of the two-week wait is always the hardest, especially those days leading up to when your period is due or when you are going to take a pregnancy test. This is when I needed to stop and breathe the most, especially every time I needed to go to the toilet, as I was absolutely terrified that I would find blood. Go shopping and treat yourself to something nice, like some new shoes or a handbag. Something that is going to make you happy and feel good.

These techniques can help to keep you occupied during the two-week wait, which can help to calm the mind and keep you a little sane. However, ultimately, there is nothing you can do to speed things up or change the outcome. You just have to wait and see. I kept saying to myself, it will happen when the time is right for me. If I get my period, it is not my time.

Chapter summary

Here are some actions you can take to implement the key points from this chapter.

1. Consider purchasing a pendulum from a crystal store and use it to seek answers from your body. If you are interested in muscle testing, you may also wish to book in with a local kinesiologist who can do a session with you to see what you need.

2. Crystals are a great low cost, support for your fertility journey. Do any of the crystals I wrote about resonate with you? Perhaps this is the crystal you need.

3. Have you told the universe about your desires for a baby? Write your goals and desires weekly to the universe, as well as expressing gratitude for what you have.

4. Are you confident in your ability to conceive a child? Positive affirmations may help to change your mindset and encourage you to believe in yourself more positively. Write down a list of affirmations that resonate with you and stick the list somewhere where you will see it regularly such as on the fridge.

5. Plan some fun, non-fertility related activities to reduce stress and act as a distraction during the dreaded two-week wait.

Conclusion

My main goal in writing this book was to show that there may always be some hope, even if you are over the age of 40 and the odds are stacked against you. I also wanted to show that I didn't miraculously get pregnant at age 43; I had been working on improving my health for a long time and I was in the best position I could be health wise. My health was better in my early 40s than it had been for most of my life, including my childhood.

I want this book to trigger a light bulb moment for readers to help them identify areas they could look into themselves if the topics I covered resonated with them. Whether this is making dietary changes, switching from folic acid to methylfolate, buying some crystals or working to reduce stress levels.

In chapter 1, I shared my story about how I overcame 10 years of secondary infertility and recurrent pregnancy loss to conceive and give birth to a healthy baby girl at age 44. This was despite being told at age 41 that my eggs were too old, and my only hope was to use a donor.

Chapter 2 introduced secondary infertility, the principal topic of this book. I discussed how it is as common as primary infertility and how postnatal depletion can be an enormous factor, especially in terms of nutrient depletion and identifying if postpartum thyroiditis could be a factor.

In chapter 3, I covered in length foods to eat regularly to nourish your body and optimise your fertility. This included key vitamins and minerals to support fertility and good food choices. I also wrote about different dietary approaches and my personal fertility diet, which was based on the principles of the Weston A Price Foundation and the GAPS Diet.

I also discussed the truth about folic acid and why it is so detrimental to fertility for people who have the MTHFR gene mutation, and why methylfolate is so important. I also shared a little about my journey and what to do if you want to get tested to see if you have the MTHFR gene mutation.

Hippocrates said over 2000 years ago that "All diseases begin in the gut" so chapter four was always going to be a key chapter covering how digestion affects fertility. I offered insight on how to support your gut, the connection between gluten and infertility, the GAPS diet, my gut health story and immune related fertility issues.

Chapter 5 was all about hormones and how to achieve healthy hormone harmony. I looked at issues such as estrogen dominance, the impact of stress on healthy hormone balance, supporting progesterone levels and promoting healthy ovulation.

In chapter 6, I considered the issue of trying to get pregnant over the age of 40 and what the chances are statistically. I also looked at improving egg quality and the importance of boron, coenzyme Q10 and alpha lipoic acid to support fertility and mitochondrial health over the age of 40.

In chapter 7, I highlighted how stress or HPA axis dysfunction could be affecting your ability to conceive. This included nutrients to support the adrenal glands, targeted supplements, and how meditation and just taking time out to breathe can be helpful.

The focus of chapter 8 was on the thyroid gland and how both hypothyroidism and hyperthyroidism can affect fertility and may be a factor with recurrent pregnancy loss. I talked about testing, checking your basal body temperature and how to support the thyroid with essential nutrients.

In chapter 9, I explained how silent, low-grade inflammation can be a common factor in infertility and can increase the risk of autoimmune diseases. I looked at foods and nutrients that support a more balanced immune system, enhancing T reg production and reducing Th17 production, which helps to calm down inflammation and reduce the risk of autoimmunity.

The focus of chapter 10 was recurrent chemical pregnancies, which was my main issue during my fertility journey. I talked about my story of having over 17 chemical pregnancies over a 10-year period, what chemical pregnancies are, the main causes and the connection with the immune system.

It wouldn't be a complete book on unexplained secondary infertility without a chapter specifically addressing our dads to be. In chapter 11, I discussed male infertility and the common factors that are contributing to poor sperm health and low sperm count.

Chapter 12, the final chapter, was all about taking the time to listen to your body. I talked about muscle testing, how I used crystals for support, the importance of positive affirmations and regularly telling the universe about your baby dreams. I also covered the importance of beliefs and what you believe about your health and ability to get pregnant. Could your negative beliefs about your body be holding you back?

Finally, I also discussed the dreaded two-week wait and the coping mechanisms I used to get through this highly stressful waiting period.

The next step

It is important to remember that we are all individual and there is not one dietary approach or supplement regime that suits everyone, so I recommend working with a functional medicine practitioner, naturopath or fertility nutritionist to help personalise your approach depending on your needs.

If you are considering working with me, you can contact me for a FREE 15-minute consultation in the first instance over Zoom to discuss your situation and how I may be able to help you. Consultations are not available for people in the USA or Canada, unfortunately, due to insurance restrictions. I also have a small Facebook group you can join called *Optimising Fertility with Nutrition and Lifestyle Support* where you can keep in contact with me. There is also a forum to ask questions.

I hope that by reading this book, you at least feel a renewed sense of optimism that there are things you can do and work on outside the standard recommendations from your GP and fertility clinic. Nature can provide us with so much wonderful support if we allow it to. From my experience, I know that the standard medical approach can leave you feeling hopeless, especially if you have received a diagnosis of unexplained infertility.

I would love to hear if this book has helped you in any way, so please get in touch and share your story.

About the author

C atherine Garney is a registered clinical nutritionist and a certified GAPS practitioner. She runs a private practice based in Tauranga in New Zealand called Nutrition for Health, which she established in 2012. Catherine consults with clients both in person in Tauranga and online from all over New Zealand and internationally.

Catherine's area of specialisation and interest is gut health, children's health, and fertility nutrition. She has two children: a boy aged 15 and a 5-year-old girl who have their own dietary challenges, so keeps her very busy.

In 2015, Catherine was fortunate enough to attend a two-day GAPS practitioner training in Sydney with Dr. Natasha Campbell McBride, who is the author of the books *Gut and Psychology Syndrome* and *Gut and Physiology Syndrome*. It was at this course that she trained to be a certified GAPS practitioner and has, for the last 9 years, been helping clients with the GAPS nutritional protocol.

Catherine's interest in fertility comes from her own heart-breaking journey with unexplained secondary infertility and recurrent pregnancy loss. After 10 years of secondary infertility, Catherine conceived naturally and gave birth to a healthy baby girl at age 44 against the odds. After a failed IVF at age 41, her fertility doctor told her the devastating news that her eggs were too old, and her only hope was to use a donor. This left her determined to go within and literally turn herself inside out to try to work out what was wrong. Nutrition and gut healing played a big part in this journey, so Catherine created this book as a useful resource to benefit others.

Catherine's extensive knowledge about fertility, gained over the last 10 years, motivates her to help others experiencing infertility, particularly secondary infertility. Her area of focus is preconception care for both females and males and investigating unexplained and secondary infertility holistically. Catherine can help you investigate important areas that may be out of the scope of practice for your doctor. This may include nutrition, lifestyle, natural remedies, environment, mindset, stress management, addressing hormone imbalances, supporting gut health, and reducing toxicity.

For further information and resources visit: www.nutritionforhealthnz.com or you can email: catherine@nutritionforhealthnz.com. You can also follow her on social media: facebook.com/nutritionforhealthnz and Instragram.com/nutritionforhealthnz

References

Chapter 2 – Secondary infertility

1. Mascarenhas M N et al. *National, Regional and Global Trends in Infertility Prevalence since 1990: A Systemic Analysis of 277 Health Surveys*. Plos Med, 2012, Dec: 9 (12): e1001356. PubMed Dec 18, 2012

2. Woulfe C .*Revealed: how C section Scar Defects Can Cause Infertility*. 13 Aug 2018. Article sourced from: https://thespinoff.co.nz/society/13-08-2018/reve aled-how-c-section-scar-defects-can-cause-infertility

3. Ahamed F M. *Link Between Caesarean Section Scar Defect and Secondary Infertility: Case Reports and Review*. 30 Mar 2023. JBRA Assist Reprod. Vol 27 (1) 134- 141

4. Dougherty A .*C Sections Can Cause Infertility, Kiwi Mum Warns* – 16 August 2018. Sourced from: www.stuff.co.nz/life-style/parenting/conception/10631 0466/csections-can-cause-infertility-kiwi-mum-warns

5. Buening B. et al (2017) *Relationship between Pregnancy and Development of Autoimmune Diseases*. J Womens Health, Issues Care Vol 6 Issue 1. 21.1.2017

6. Serrallach O. *The Postnatal Depletion Cure: A Complete Guide to Rebuilding Your Health and Reclaiming Your Energy for Mothers of Newborns, Toddlers, and Young Children*. Hachette Australia, 2018

7. Cabot S. *Your Thyroid Problems Solved, Holistic Solutions to Improve your Thyroid*. WHAS Pty Ltd, 2006 p 67

8. Cabot S. *Your Thyroid Problems Solved, Holistic Solutions to Improve your Thyroid*. WHAS Pty Ltd, 2006 p 68

9. Verma I, Sood R, Juneja S, Kaur S. *Prevalence of Hypothyroidism in Infertile Women and Evaluation of Response of Treatment for Hypothyroidism on Infertility*. International Journal of Applied and Basic Medical Research Jan – June 2012: 2(1):17-19

Chapter 3 - Nutrition

1. Grzechocinska B, Dabroski FA, Cyganek A, Wielgus M. *The role of Vitamin D in Impaired Fertility Treatment*. Neuroendocrinology Letters, 2013 Vol 34, No 8, 756–62

2. Lerchbaum E, Rabe T. *Vitamin D and Female Fertility*. Current Opinion in Obstetrics and Gynecology. June 2014, 26(3) 145 -50

3. Servy E J et al. *MTHFR isoform carriers. 5-MTHF (5-methyltetrahydrofolate) vs folic acid: a key to pregnancy outcomes: a case series*. Journal of Assisted Reproduction and Genetics. 7 June 2018, Vol 35 (8):1431-1435

4. Lynch Dr Ben. *Dirty Genes* ,2018, P 48, Harper One

5. Gray N. *Could Active Folate boost IVF chances. Fertility Study backs 5-MTFHR over Folic acid* -www.nutraingredients.com/article/2018/07/13

6. Erum A, et al. *Association of Plasma Folic Acid, Vitamin B12 and Homocysteine with Recurrent Pregnancy Loss*. "A Case Control Study" Pak J Med Sci, 2023, Sept–Oct 39 (5) 1280–1285

7. Pacholok S M (13/12/2013) *Vitamin B12 Deficiency: Serious Consequences* – Pharmacy Times, December 2013, Vol 79, Issue 12

8. Kresser C (6/5/2011) *B12 Deficiency: A Silent Epidemic with Serious Consequences* – sourced from www.chrisresser.com

Additional resources:

• The Weston A Price Foundation. *Timeless Principles of Healthy Traditional Diets. Wise Traditions. Sourced 2023*

Chapter 4 – Gut health

1. Bold J, Rostami K. *Non-Coeliac Gluten Sensitivity and Reproductive Disorders.* Autumn 2015. Vol 8 (4) 294 -297. Sourced from: www.ncbi.nlm.nih.gov

2. Choi Janet M, et al. *Increased Prevalence of Coeliac Disease in Patients with Unexplained Infertility in the United States*: A Prospective Study. Journal of Reproductive Medicine. May – June 2011, (56) 5-6: 199–203

3. Tersigni C, et al. *Coeliac Disease and Reproductive Disorder: Meta-Analysis of Epidemiologic Associations and Potential Pathogenic Mechanisms.* Human Reproduction Update, 2014. Vol 20 No 4 582–593

4. Casella G et al. *Coeliac Disease and Obstetrical-Gynecological Contribution.* Gastroenterol Hepatol Bed Bench, Fall 2016. Vol 9, Issue 4 241-249

5. Ferguson R, Holmes G K, Louke W. *Coeliac Disease, Fertility and Pregnancy,* Scand J Gastroenterol. Jan 1982. Vol 17, issue 1, 65–68

6. Grode L, et al. *Reproductive Life in Women with Coeliac Disease; a Nationwide Population-Based Matched Cohort Study.* June 15, 2018. Human Reproduction, Vol 33, No 8 1538-1547

7. Larsen J et al. *Dietary Gluten Increases Natural Killer Cell Cytotoxicity and Cytokine Secretion.* European Journal of Immunology, 10 July 2014. Vol 44, 3056 -3067

Additional resources:

- Campbell-McBride Dr N MD, *Gut and Psychology Syndrome*, 2015, Medinform

- Campbell- McBride D N MD, *Gut and Physiology Syndrome*, 2020, Medinform

- Fallon S, *Nourishing Traditions*, 1999, New Trends Publishing.

Chapter 5 – Hormone harmony

1. Romm A, MD. *The Estrobolome: The Fascinating Way Your Gut Impacts your Estrogen Levels*, 14th April 2021, www.avivaromm.com/estrobolome

2. Kresser C *How Gut Microbes Influence Estrogen Levels*, 15th Nov 2017, sourced from: www.kresserinstitute.com/gut-hormone-connection-gut-microbiome-influence-estrogen-levels

3. Oyelowo T, *Mosby's Guide to Women's Health*, 2007, p 8 – 10, Elsevier Inc.

4. Joseph DN, Whirledge S. *Stress and the HPA Axis: Balancing Homeostasis and Fertility.* International Journal of Molecular Sciences, Oct 24, 2017, 18 (10) 2224

5. Medline Plus. *SHBG Blood test* – sourced from Medlineplus.govllab-tests/SHBG-blood-test (14/12/22)

6. Brighten Dr. J. *Low Testosterone in Women and How to Increase T Naturally.* 18 Dec 2022. Sourced from: www.drbrighten.com/low-testosterone-in-women

7. Chandrasekhar K et al. *A Prospective, Randomized Double-Blind, Placebo-Controlled Study of Safety and Efficacy of a High-Concentration Full-Spectrum Extract of Ashwagandha Root in Reducing Stress and Anxiety in Adults.* Indian J Psychol Med, 2012 July- Sept, 34 (3) 255- 262

8. Tyrakithanakan et al. *Effects of Mindfulness Meditation on Serum Cortisol of Medical Studies.* J Med Assoc, Thai, 2013 Jan 96, Suppl 1:590-5

9. Brighten Dr. J. *Low Testosterone in Women and How to Increase T Naturally.* 18 Dec 2022. Sourced from: www.drbrighten.com/low-testosterone-in-women

10. Jean Hailes for Women's Health, article on Fibroids. 29th June 2021. Sourced from: www.jeanhailes.org.au/health-a-z/ovaries-uterus/fibroids

11. Hajhshemi M MD et al. *The Effect of vitamin D Supplementation on the Size of Uterine Leiomyoma in Women with Vitamin D Deficiency.* Caspian J Intern Med, 2019 Spring 10 (2) 125 - 131

Additional resources:

• Esche-Belke S, Kircschner-Brouns. *Our Hormones, Our Health: How to Understand your Hormones and Transform Your Life*, 2021, Scribe Publications

Chapter 6 - Fertility over 40

1. American Society of Reproductive Medicine, *Age and Fertility Booklet-* sourced from www.reproductivefacts.org/news-and-publications/fact-sheets-and-info graphics/age-and-fertility-booklet (sourced June 2023)

2. Extend Fertility – Fertility Statistics by Age. Sourced from: www.extendfertili ty.com/your-fertility/fertility-stats-by-age (sourced June 2023)

3. Brim E. S MD. *Getting Pregnant at 40, FAQS and Tip for Optimising your Fertility Health.* Virginia Physicians for Women. www.wpfw.com (9/11/23)

4. Yangying Xu et al. *Pretreatment with Coenzyme Q10 Improves Ovarian Response and Embryo Quality in Low Prognosis Young Women with Decreased Ovarian Reserve: A Randomised Controlled Trial.* Reprod Biol Endocrinol, 27th March 2018. Vol 16: 29

5. Know Lee ND. *Mitochondria and the Future of Medicine.* Charles Green Publishing, 2018

6. Benkhalifa M et al. *Mitochondrial Participation to Infertility as a Source of Energy and cause of Senescence,* Int. J. Biochem. Cell. Biol 2014. 55: 60-64

7. Tatone C et al. *Age-Dependent Changes in the Expression of Superoxide Dismutase and Catalase are associated with Ultrastructural Modification in Human Granulosa Cells.* Mol. Hum. Reprod 2006: 12 655-666

8. Fett R, *It Starts with the Egg.* Second Edition, 2019, Franklin Fox Publishing

9. Kim C et al. *Lipoic Acid Supplementation Increases the Expression of Pgc-1 Alpha Gene in Granuosa Cells and Improves IVF results in Aging Women Undergoing IVF.* September 2017. Fertility and Sterility, Vol 108, issue 3, supplement E228. Sourced from: www.fertstart.org/article/S0015-0282 (17) 31211-6/fulltext

10. Haghighlan H K et al. *Randomised Triple-blind, Placebo Controlled Clinical Trial Examines the Effects of Alpha Lipoic Acid Supplementation on the Spermatogonium and Seminal Oxidative Stress in the Infertile Male.* August 2015. Fertility and Sterility. Vol 104 (2): 318-24

11. Forrest F H (PHD) and Meacham S L (PHD). May 9th, 2011. *Growing Evidence for Human Health Benefits of Boron,* Journal of Evidence-Based Complementary and Alternative Medicine. Vol 16 (3) 169 -180

12. Levy J. Boron Uses – *Boost Bone Density and Much* More. 12th September 2020. sourced from: www.draxe.com/nutrition/boronuses

13. Levy J. *Boron Uses – Boost Bone Density and Much More.* 12th September 2020. Sourced from: www.draxe.com/nutrition/boronuses

14. Forrest F H (PHD) and Meacham S L (PHD). May 9th, 2011. *Growing Evidence for Human Health Benefits of Boron,* Journal of Evidence-Based Complementary and Alternative Medicine. Vol 16 (3) 169 -180

Chapter 7 – Stress

1. Kalantaridou S N et al. *Stress and the Female Reproductive System.* June 2004. J Reprod Immunol. Vol 62 (1-2) 61–8

2. Jimena P et al. *Adrenal Hormones in Human Follicular Fluid.* Acta Endocrinol, Nov 1992, Issue 127 (5): 403-6. Sourced from: www.pubmed.ncbi/nlm.nih.gov/1471451 (sourced Dec 2023)

3. Mas Bagüés C, *Geoscience, a Unifying View on Aging as a Risk Factor.* 23rd Sept 2022. Aging: from Fundamental Biology to Societal Impact – sourced from www.sciencedirect.com/science/articles/abs/pii/B9780128237618000288

Additional resources:

• World Health Organisation (WHO). Burnout definition. Sourced From: www.who.int/news/item/28-05-2019-burn-out-an-occupational-phenomenon-international-classification-of-disease. Sourced: Feb 2024

Chapter 8 – Thyroid dysfunction

1. Mazokopakis EE et al. *Is vitamin D Related to Pathogenesis and Treatment of Hashimoto's thyroiditis.* Sept-Dec 2015. Hellenic Journal of Nuclear Medicine. Vol 18 (3) 222-7

2. Messina M et al. *Neither Soy Foods nor Isoflavones Warrant Classification as Endocrine Disruptors: a Technical Review of the Observational and Clinical Data.* Critical Review Food Science Nutrition. March 2021. Vol 62 (21): 5824–85

3. *Myers A MD. The Autoimmune Solution: Prevent and Reverse the Full Spectrum of Inflammatory Symptoms and Diseases.* 2015. Harper One

4. Benvenga S et al. *Effects of Carnitine on Thyroid Hormone Action*. Annals of the New York Academy of Sciences. November 2004. 1033:158-67

Chapter 9 – Inflammation

1. Ehsani M et al. *Female Unexplained Infertility: A Disease with Imbalanced Adaptive Immunity*. Journal of Human Reproductive Sciences, Oct - Dec 2019, p 275

2. Oukka M et al. *Th17 Cells in Immunity and Autoimmunity*. Dec 2008. *BMJ Journal, Annals of Rheumatic Disease*, Vol 67, suppl 3, 26-9

3. Ehsani M et al. *Female Unexplained Infertility: A Disease with Imbalanced Adaptive Immunity*. Journal of Human Reproductive Sciences, Oct-Dec 2019, p 276

4. Rocamera-Reverte et al. 27 Jan 2021. *The Complex Role of Regulatory T Cells in Immunity and Aging*. Immunol, Vol 11, Frontiers in Nutrition

5. Jian Tan et al. *Your Regulatory T Cells are What You Eat. How Diet and Gut Microbiome Affect Regulatory T Cell Development*. 20 April 2022. Frontiers in Nutrition. 20:9:878382

6. Siddiqui MT et al. *The Immunomodulatory Functions of Butyrate*. Nov 18 2021. J Inflamm Res. Vol 14: 6025-6041

7. Liu L et al., *Butyrate Interferes with the Differentiation and Function of Human Monocyte – Derived Dendritic Cells*. May-June 2012. Cell Immunol 277 (1-2) 66–73

8. Ho E, *Mechanisms Discovered for Health Benefits of Green Tea, New Approaches to Autoimmune Disease*. 3 June 2021. Oregon State University. www.scienced aily.com/releases/2011/06/110602143214.htm

9. Fisher S A et al. *The Role of Vitamin D in Increasing Circulating T Regulatory Cells*, 24 Sept 2019. PLos One. Sourced from: https://pubmed.ncbi.nlm.nih .gov/31550254/

10. Ross A C. *Vitamin A and Retinoic Acid in T Cell Related Immunity*. Nov 2012. AMJ Clinical Nutrition. Vol 96 (5) 11665-11725

11. Hsien-Yeh Hsu et al. *Reishi Protein Induces FOXP3+ T Reg Expansion Via a CD45 Dependent Signalling Pathway and Alleviates Acute Intestinal Inflammation in Mice*. 24 June 2013. Evid Based Complement Alternate Med. 2013:513542. Sourced from: www.pubmed.ncbi.nlm.nih.gov/23864893/

12. Barron J. *Systemic Proteolytic Enzymes*. 27 July 2014. The Baseline of Health Foundation. Sourced from: www.jonbarron.org/article/proteolytic-enzyme-f ormula

Chapter 10 – Chemical pregnancies

1. Kuniaki et al. *Vitamin D Deficiency May be a Risk Factor for Recurrent Pregnancy Loss by Increasing Cellular Immunity and Autoimmunity*. Feb 2014. Human Reproduction, vol 29, no 2, pp 208-219

2. Leischner C, Burkard M, Pfeiffer M. *Nutritional Immunology: Function of Natural Killer Cells and their Modulation by Resveratrol for Cancer Prevention and Treatment*. 4 May 2016. Nutrition Journal 15 (1): 47

3. Gaynor LM, Colucci F. *Uterine Natural Killer Cells: Functional Distinctions and Influences in Pregnancy in Humans and Mice*. 24 April 2017. Front Immunol 24:8:467

4. McFarlin K B et al. *Oral Spore-Based Probiotic Supplementation was Associated with Reduced Incidence of Post Prandial Dietary Endotoxin, Triglycerides, and Disease Risk Biomarkers*. 15 August 2017. World Gastrointest Pathophysiol, vol 8 (3) 117-126

Additional resources:

- Wentz I, *Hashimoto's Protocol: A 90-Day Plan for Reversing Thyroid Symptoms and Getting Your Life Back*, 2016. Harper One

Chapter 11 – Male infertility

1. Hurst L. *Sperm Counts are Declining, Scientist Believe They Have Pinpointed the Main Causes Why*. 15 June 2023. Sourced from: https://www.euronews.com/health/2023/06/15/sperm-counts-are-declining-scientists-believe-they-have-pinpointed-the-main-causes-why

2. Jurkowska K et al. *The Impact of Metalloestrogens on the Physiology of Male Reproductive Health as a Current problem of the XXI Century*. 18 Sept 2019. J Physiol Pharmacol. Vol 70 (3) 337-55

3. Daniela Paes de Almeida Ferreira Braga et al. *Food Intake and Social Habits in Male Patients and its Relationship to Intracytoplasmic Sperm Injection Outcome*. Jan 2012. Fertil Steril. 97(1):53-9

4. Ahahmar A T et al. *The Impact of Two Doses of Coenzyme Q10 on Semem Parameters and Antioxidant Status in Men with Idiopathic Oligoasthenteratozoospermia*. Sept 2019. Clin Exp Reprod Med. Vol 46 (3) 112-118

5. Salas–Huetus A et al. *The Effects of Nutrients and Dietary Supplements on Sperm Quality Parameters: A Systematic Review and Meta Analysis of Randomised Clinical Trials*. Nov 2018. Advances in Nutrition, vol 9, issue 6, 883-848

6. Mateus F G et al. *L-Carnitine and Male Fertility. Is Supplementation Beneficial?* Sep 2024. J Clinic Med. Vol 6:12 (18): 5796

7. Campbell-McBride Dr N, *Gut and Physiology Syndrome.* 2020. Medinform Publishing

Chapter 12 – Listen to your body

1. Hall J. *The Crystal Bible: A Definitive Guide to Crystals*, 2003, p 235

Additional resources:

- Raupp A E. *Body Belief: How to Heal Autoimmune Diseases, Radically Shift Your Health, and Learn to Love Your Body More.* 2018. Hay House Inc

- Bernstein G. *Super Attractor: Methods for Manifesting a Life Beyond Your Wildest Dreams. 2019.* Hay House Inc

www.ingramcontent.com/pod-product-compliance
Lightning Source LLC
Chambersburg PA
CBHW072121020426
42334CB00018B/1675